ESSENTIAL FAMILY AND TRAVELLERS' HEALTH

DR. USEN IKIDDE

Copyright © 2016 Usen Ikidde

All Rights Reserved

No part of this book may be reproduced in any form by electronic or mechanical means, including information storage and retrieval systems, without permission in writing from the author or publisher, except by a reviewer who may quote brief passages in a review or by a licence permitting restricted copying.

Whilst the advice in this book is believed to be true and accurate at the date of going to press, neither the author nor the publisher can accept any legal responsibility or liability for any errors or omissions that may be made. Secondly this book does not in anywhere constitute a prescription nor a final advice which should be referred at all times to family doctors and specialist where the history can be taken and a one to one physical and psychological clinical assessment can be made.

ESSENTIAL FAMILY AND TRAVELLERS' HEALTH

DR. USEN IKIDDE

E book copies may be obtained from Amazon Kindle, kobo, nook, Sony e Reader, Apple iBooks etc.
Paper copies may be obtained from Amazon and by order from major bookshops worldwide.

This book is dedicated to my wife, Mercy, and children for their love, patience and support.

Contents

Contents 5
ACKNOWLEDGEMENTS viii
PREFACE ix
CHAPTER ONE 1
   IMMUNISATION, DISEASE PREVENTION AND
   ACTIVE IMMUNITY 1
   ACTIVE IMMUNITY 3
   IMMUNISATION SCHEDULE FROM SUMMER 2015 .. 11
CHAPTER TWO 14
   NON-ROUTINE IMMUNISATION PROGRAMME IN
   THE UK 14
   ANTHRAX 14
   BOTULISM 15
   CHOLERA 15
   HEPATITIS A 16
   JAPANESE ENCEPHALITIS 17
   RABIES 17
   SMALL POX 19
   TICK-BORNE ENCEPHALITIS 19
   TYPHOID FEVER 21
   CHICKEN POX 23
   HERPES ZOOSTER (Shingles) 27
   YELLOW FEVER 29
CHAPTER THREE 34
   PASSIVE IMMUNITY 34

- Immunoglobulin 36
- 1. HEPATITIS B 39
- 2. RABIES 40
- 3 TETANUS. 40
- 4. CHICKEN POX 41
- Rhesus Disease 44

CHAPTER FOUR 47

- DISEASE PREVENTION IN INTERNATIONAL TRAVEL 47
- 1. MALARIA 50
- 2. TUBERCULOSIS(TB) 60
- 3. YELLOW FEVER 64
- EBOLA 65
- LASSA FEVER 69
- MEASLES 73
- AFRICAN TRYPANOSOMIASIS (SLEEPING SICKNESS) 78
- BIRD FLU (AVIAN FLU) 83
- DENGUE FEVER 86
- HAND, FOOT AND MOUTH DISEASE 97
- LEPTOSPIROSIS 103
- MENINGOCOCCAL DISEASE (Meningococcus) 108
- MURRAY VALLEY ENCEPHALITIS VIRUS 113
- PNEUMOCOCCAL DISEASE (Streptococcus pneumonia) 116
- RABIES 121
- RIFT VALLEY FEVER 125
- SCHISTOSOMIASIS (bilharzia) 133
- TETANUS 139

- MIDDLE EAST RESPIRATORY SYNDROME (MERS) 150
- SARS (Severe Acute Respiratory Syndrome) 155
- ZIKA VIRUS 159
- CHAPTER FIVE 166
  - SEXUALLY TRANSMITTED DISEASES (STD) - 166
  - CHLAMYDIA 168
  - GENITAL WARTS 175
  - GENITAL HERPIS 178
  - GONORRHOEA 181
  - SYPHILIS 185
  - HUMAN IMMUNODEFFICIENCY VIRUS (HIV) 193
  - TRICHOMONIASIS 203
  - PUBIC LICE (Pediculosis pubis or Phthirus) 206
  - SCABIES 208
  - HEPATITIS B VIRUS 213
  - PELVIC INFLAMMATORY DISEASE (PID) 222
  - LYMPHOGRANULOMA VENEREUM (LGV) 227
  - CHANCROID 229
  - MOLLUSCUM CONTAGIOSUM 232
- CHAPTER SIX 237
  - NEGLECTED TROPICAL DISEASEs 237
- REFERENCES 241

ACKNOWLEDGEMENTS

1. My wife, Mercy, who showed great patience and understanding during the writing of this book.
2. Dr.Ema Etuknwa who diligently read the manuscript.

PREFACE

This book is intended for the family and travellers, some of who do not pay much attention to several diseases and infections which are truly preventable. The old age adage that "prevention is better than cure" holds true today even more than what it was several years ago.

More infections and diseases which were either unknown or did not exist are coming to the attention of doctors and the public at large. Human civilization and air travel have brought the world into what has aptly been described as "a global village".

Whilst such interactions in trade, cooperation, friendship and leisure have been of immense benefit to the human race, there have also been a few disadvantages: the spread of hitherto unknown infections which we were either unaware of, or have paid little or no attention as to their importance, and their enormity are coming into focus.

Our awareness of these diseases, virulence, spread and prevention are important aspects of this book. It is a compendium of such infections, recognition, prevention and management outlines, but does not constitute a prescription or final advice which can only be given in a clinical setting.

We cannot take care of things we don't know or know very little about or sometimes have only heard them mentioned in passing and conclude that they don't concern us. When that happens we often pay very little or no attention to their importance because we assume that they are not for us and their significance are therefore downgraded or completely disregarded.

"Knowledge is power". We need the knowledge to control our environment, infections, diseases and plan how to prevent them. Without knowledge, we cannot act and that is what this book is all about-the acquisition of knowledge to help us manage, plan and prevent diseases and infections.

On the other hand when we realize that something concerns us, we tend to pay more attention to it and treat such matter with the importance and significance it deserves. That is the case with infections and their prevention.

It is easy enough to say that we are never going to travel to other parts of the world where such infections are prevalent or endemic but we do not live in isolation. We have families, friends, acquaintances, co-workers, hosts, visitors or guests and these are important routes of transmission of infections and diseases. Human- human contacts form important routes of transmission of infections. That means that we don't have to visit endemic or pandemic regions of the world to become candidates: we only need to have a family member, a friend or co-worker or sometimes a casual meeting with someone to pick up certain infections.

The prevention is not to avoid all human contacts because that is impossible. Even if we did that, what of the vectors, food, articles, water, unforeseen circumstances like flooding, the air we breathe or our pets etc?

The solution often lies not only in avoidance but in recognition and adoption of preventive measures including immunization. The latter is the sin qua non where practicable as it is the most important means of prevention in addition to other measures which are clearly stated in this book.

The importance of prevention in medicine is underpinned by the emphasis placed on immunization and immunization programmes and schedules set out in this book. Timing and completion of immunization programmes are important to ensure immunity and protection. Childhood immunization is particularly important because healthy children become healthy and health-conscious adults.

Non-scheduled immunization apply to certain groups particularly travellers and susceptibility due to age or sex related infections which may lead to serious health problems. The book therefore tries to cover all aspects as far as possible and so there are a few exceptions which should also be borne in mind when taking up vaccination or immunization.

Distinction is made between active and passive immunization. The former helps the body to produce its own natural defence-antibodies which fight infections whereas in the latter the antibodies have already been produced and can be injected immediately especially in life-threatening conditions. That is the main advantage of passive immunization, namely: urgency and speed of action.

Active immunization, though lacking these elements, has the advantage of longevity of action and in some cases greater efficiency and effectiveness. It is therefore preferred to passive immunization in circumstances where speed of action is not an important factor or where immunization is a long term goal rather than a medical emergency. In certain circumstances, a combination of both could offer the best solution so that whilst passive immunization protects immediately, active immunization takes over and offers long term protection.

The importance of prevention and immunization against infections during international travel has for long been neglected or not given the proper priority it deserves. The result is that preventable infections have not been immunized against or contact prevented by adopting adequate and effective measures resulting in infections which should have been prevented.

With development of faster means of transport, especially the aeroplane, the world has become one "global village". With improvement in standard of living, wages, knowledge, better and faster means of transport and man's natural propensity to expand horizons, explore other cultures or take well deserved vacations/ holidays abroad, there has been a marked increase in communication and air travel. Whilst this has been very advantageous both for the individual and the transport industry, there have also been a few disadvantages and downside: the speed which infectious diseases can be carried across borders. It is now possible to traverse from Los Angeles, New York, London, Paris, Moscow, Rome, Cairo, Lagos, Tokyo, Sydney, Delhi, Beijing within days. That is the same speed and duration in which infectious and communicable diseases travel.

The trans-national, transoceanic and global nature of infections, which at its worst may be the harbinger of epidemics and pandemics have been emphasized in this book. The lessons we have learnt from Ebola and Zika viruses should open our eyes to the realities of epidemics and pandemics.

Sexually transmitted infections (STI) especially HIV is another case in point. The widespread or global transmission has been no respecter of national or international boundaries. The author has therefore decided to look at STI from different angles, namely: purely as STI and secondly from a traveller's perspective. Some other infections have been approached from these two or multi-perspective dimensions. To this end such infections have been discussed in more than one area to cover all interests.

The World Health Organization, WHO, has recently drawn the world's attention to "Neglected Tropical Diseases"(NTD) which should require no further expatiation and explanation at this stage as the name speaks for itself and aptly justifies its choice. The importance of NTD has been rightly underpinned by the significance and emphasis given to it that Bill Gates and his wife, Melinda, have not only helped in justifying the importance of NTD verbally but by putting their financial resources in the establishment of Bill and Melinda Gates Foundation.

The importance of NTD is dealt with comprehensively in the last chapter of this book.

This book is an essential read for every family, traveller and visitor to other regions and countries worldwide. Endemic and holo-endemic regions of most known or less well known infections are highlighted and emphasized. To make it readable to the layman, which this work is mostly intended, explanations of most of the medical terms are given in brackets.

It is important to point out that medical students and doctors of all grades especially those who have had little or no exposure to Tropical Medicine and Public Health are also encouraged to read this book.

Dr. Usen Ikidde

Lastly, whilst discouraging complacency, it is also important to state that we are not being invaded by unknown bacteria and viruses as most of these infections have been known to exist before any epidemic or pandemic occurred. What has been lacking in most cases is the knowledge and thus the need for preventive measures. This author has made such knowledge and understanding available to everyone. Truly, "knowledge is power" and that power lies within us. We do not have knowledge without access to it and having access requires knowledge.

CHAPTER ONE

IMMUNISATION, DISEASE PREVENTION AND ACTIVE IMMUNITY.

There is no doubt that "prevention is better than cure". This is true not only in terms of resources, human and financial, accidents and even relationships but also the uncertainty of a cure after contracting a disease or illness which could easily have been prevented but if it becomes established there is potential for morbidity (illness) and mortality (death). Prevention does not only apply to disease prevention but in virtually all human endeavours and situations in life especially in our jobs, financial matters and intimate and not so intimate relationships. There are unpleasant situations in life which with the benefits of hindsight we could have prevented but had not done so. Often we ignore mental illness as totally out of the reach of prevention; that is not the case as many types of mental health problems are preventable and even those that are not purely so, respond better to early intervention.

Let us now turn our attention to disease prevention. How do we prevent disease? The first and very important aspect is the prevention of contact with communicable, contagious and infectious diseases. There is no point in coming into contact with someone infected with, say, Ebola virus, without all the necessary preventive measures and if there is no need to be there at all in the vicinity, then why go there? Health care professionals who have a duty to treat patients with Ebola must ensure that they take all necessary measures and precautions to prevent being infected. Other highly infectious diseases like tuberculosis, flu, chicken pox, whooping cough, measles and insect transmitted diseases or infections fall into the same category.

Immunisation (inoculation or vaccination) is one of the most important aspects of disease prevention. These terms all refer to the same process whereby attenuated or inactive or dead micro organisms are introduced into the body usually by injection or orally as in polio. The attenuated or inactive organisms then stimulate the body's immune system to produce antibodies to fight that particular disease either immediately or if that disease recurs in the future.

Immunisation, (vaccination or inoculation) remains the bedrock for the prevention of infectious diseases especially in childhood. To this end, a schedule of immunisation should be followed and adhered to. Most children and adults derive considerable benefit by sticking to and having immunisation at the stipulated times. The schedule or timing usually takes into consideration the age of the child or adult and the age of their possible susceptibility to a number of these infections. In some cases, immunisation is given as a result of contact with an infected individual or when there has been a cluster of infection when certain individuals in the susceptible age group or gender are more likely to be infected.

There are two main types of vaccine-those that provide active or passive immunisation. Active immunity can also be acquired by individuals who have already been infected by the particular disease. Active vaccines stimulate the production of antibodies and other components against the particular disease. It follows therefore that active vaccines can not usually be given to effect immediate cure except in circumstances where there is no possible alternative, in which case other measures such as antiviral or antibiotics should be given as well whilst waiting for the vaccine to take over.

Passive vaccine on the other hand usually gives immediate immunity and protection to fight the intended infection. They are normally obtained from the plasma of immune individuals with adequate levels of antibody to counteract the disease for which the protection is sought. They are usually in the form of immunoglobulins obtained from human subjects; when obtained from animals it is referred to as antisera. Antisera may give rise to serum sickness and other allergic reactions. They are therefore now rarely used. The use of immunoglobulins from human subjects is the preferred option. Immunity conferred by passive immunisation is usually temporary as the immunity lasts for a short time only; usually a few weeks and a repeat immunisation may be necessary.

ACTIVE IMMUNITY.

There are several types or preparations of active immunisation:

1. Active immunization can be acquired by natural disease which produces antibodies and when we come into contact with the same disease or infection next time , the antibodies fight the infection. In such cases where immunity has been acquired naturally, no artificial vaccination is required as immunity has already been established due to previous contact with the virus or bacteria. It is important to note that as a result of this immunity, immunoglobulin from such individuals can be used to produce "inactive" vaccine. Such inactive vaccine may also be produced from individuals who have been vaccinated with active vaccine and immunity has sufficiently been acquired and so their immunoglobulin

becomes useful as passive vaccine to people who need immunity or treatment of infection urgently.

2. Active immunisation can also be acquired artificially by injection of vaccine which may be prepared in the following ways:

   a. **Inactivated preparation of the virus or bacteria** and because it is inactivated it lacks the potential to cause infection. This is the case in influenza vaccine.
   b. **A live attenuated form of the virus or bacteria** but because it is attenuated or weakened, the potential to cause infection is equally weakened. This is the case with MMR (Measles, Mumps, Rubella vaccines which are either provided individually or preferably combined to ensure high population take up of this immunization and the important benefits) The bacterial vaccine of tuberculosis or BCG is prepared in the same way- live attenuated form of the bacteria.
   c. **A detoxified exotoxins** which is the product of micro-organism as in tetanus vaccine.
   d. Active vaccine may also be derived from **extracts of micro-organism** derived from the organism as in pneumococcal vaccine.
   e. Sometimes **a recombinant DNA technology** is used to produce an active vaccine as in hepatitis B vaccine.

Natural infection or immunity acquired in this manner produces the best long lasting immunity and a live attenuated vaccine is second best as it also produces immunity that lasts for a long period of time.

However, natural infection as a means of acquiring active immunity is not encouraged purely for this purpose as the eventual outcome is uncertain. It may result in severe complications, disability or death. Therefore natural active immunity should be by accident, not by design as the eventual outcome of the latter is virtually unpredictable.

Vaccination may usually be postponed if the would- be recipient is suffering with an acute illness especially if accompanied by fever and systemic illness.

Vaccination should not be given to individuals with a known history of anaphylactic reaction(severe allergic reaction) to a previous dose of the same vaccine. It is important for patient and physician to have a record, a warning or alert to prevent giving the individual the particular vaccine.

The manufacture of certain vaccines involves the use of **egg**. For this reason, individuals who are **allergic to eggs** should not be given such vaccines. The vaccines include **yellow fever** vaccine, **tick-borne encephalitis** vaccine and **influenza vaccine**. These vaccines may sometimes be given under specialist supervision in an emergency where there is no possible alternative. This usually involves prophylactic (preventive) or anti- anaphylactic measures - pre, during and post injection. It is a delicate balancing act between the possibility of overwhelming infection and the potential anaphylactic reaction.

Live vaccines should also be avoided, at least, temporarily in people who are immunosuppressed (very low immunity to infections) This is because such individuals could develop a generalised infection if given live vaccine. Secondly, immune response may be reduced in such people and therefore unwise and of no benefit to give any vaccination when they cannot adequately produce antibodies to fight infection because of their impaired immunity.

Patients who are on prolonged periods of high dose steroid generally have low immunity. Such patients should therefore not be given active immunization as immunosuppression by steroid poses a problem due to their inability to produce antibodies and as noted above there is a risk of generalised infection if given live attenuated vaccine.

There is also a problem with patients who are on chemotherapy or generalised radiotherapy for malignancy (cancer). Such patients also tend to have a suppressed immunity and therefore an impaired immune response.

It is considered that in certain conditions like infection due to rotavirus, the benefit of vaccination may outweigh the risks.

Generally, the specialist should be consulted in immunosuppressed individuals as in some cases the benefit may outweigh the risks and in others the degree of immunodeficiency or compromise may be judged as not sufficient to deny vaccination which may be more beneficial despite the small risk involved.

There is a theoretical risk of fetal infection in pregnancy and routine administration of live vaccine is therefore not advocated. However, in some cases the risk of infection outweighs the small risk of fetal infection. In cases such as yellow fever, it is usually recommended by the specialist to give vaccination.

It should be noted that the restrictions apply to live vaccines only: the use of inactivated viral or bacterial vaccines or toxoids are therefore usually considered to be safe though specific exclusions may sometimes apply and expert advice should be sought where there are any doubts.

There is also a theoretical risk of giving live attenuated vaccine to breast-feeding mothers as infection could be transmitted to the baby in the milk. Generally, however, the benefits of vaccinating outweigh the risk especially in well known situations where the mother has been exposed to a life-threatening infection.

HIV positive patients require specific consideration. Such patients should receive mumps, measles and rubella vaccines (MMR)normally except in severe immune impairment.

The same principle applies to vaccination against chickenpox (varicella-zoster vaccine)and rota virus.

HIV patients should not be denied the inactivated vaccines-anthrax, cholera (oral), hepatitis A & B, diphtheria, haemophilus influenzae type b, human papillomavirus, meningococcal, pertussis, pneumococcal, poliomyelitis, tetanus, rabies, typhoid (injection) and tick-borne encephalitis vaccines.

The following vaccines are however contraindicated in HIV patients(should not receive):

- BCG,
- typhoid (oral),
- yellow fever,
- influenza nasal spray except in stable cases and those on antiretroviral therapy) and
- live oral poliomyelitis vaccine as this may rarely cause vaccine-associated paralytic polio.

There are occasional side effects of vaccination which one should bear in mind. Vaccine injection may give rise to local reactions such as redness of the area, pain and inflammation. Occasionally an abscess may develop at the injection site. There may also be other symptoms which may be experienced beyond the injection site. There may be loss of appetite, fever, headache, irritability,and muscle pain.

Less common side effects include dizziness, pins and needles sensation, flu-like symptoms, drowsiness, rashes, joint pain, and enlarged lymph nodes.

Hypersensitivity reactions may very rarely occur and include asthma-like symptoms such as bronchospasm. Uticaria,angioedema, and anaphylaxis may also occur.

Oral vaccines(cholera, live oral poliomyelitis, rotavirus, and live typhoid) may also cause direct gastrointestinal symptoms including nausea, vomiting, diarrhoea, cramps and abdominal pains.

Live attenuated vaccines -Mumps, Measles and Rubella (MMR) have been known to cause very mild forms of the diseases occasionally.

In the infant, if fever develops after immunisation, the child should be given paracetamol to help lower the temperature and this can be given after every 4-6 hours.Ibuprofen is an alternative which may also be combined with paracetamol but Ibuprofen should be given 3 times daily.If fever persists, parents should seek medical help not only for post immunisation pyrexia(fever) but for the fact that the fever may be due to some other medical problem which was not immediately obvious.

Post immunisation pyrexia may complicate febrile convulsions in a child with a personal or family history of convulsions. There is a higher risk of convulsions occurring in a child who is prone to febrile convulsions. However, it is not usually considered a contraindication to immunise children with a family history of febrile convulsions unless there had previously been neurological complications following an episode of febrile convulsion. The child can also be given paracetamol or Ibuprofen as preventive measures before immunisation.

Premature(Preterm) babies require special consideration. Nonetheless, they should be immunised based on their actual date of birth not on the date they should have been born, had there not been born early. There is an increase in breathing problems which is worse in those born before 28 weeks of pregnancy. It is recommended that the risk of breathing problems are better dealt with if immunisation is undertaken in hospital rather than at home. Any problems that arise such as breathing problems, low heart rate or poor oxygen saturation are better dealt with in the hospital environment where the child should be monitored for at least 48 hours. If any of the problems occurred, it is also recommended that the second vaccine should be given in hospital.

There could be the problem of antibody production in the very premature babies less than 28 weeks of gestation. The same problem may also be encountered in babies on steroids for chronic lung disease.

Testing for antibodies to certain infections(Haemophilus influenzae type b, meningococcal C and hepatitis B) is usually recommended after the first (primary) immunisation.

Immunisation schedule takes into consideration the age of the child or adult and when the particular infections are likely to occur. It also considers the immunisation for those outside these ages but considered to be at risk. It

Dr. Usen Ikidde

follows therefore that the 2 most important considerations are age and risk factors.

Immunization schedule below applies mostly to the United Kingdom but may also be adopted, extended or modified for most other countries. It has been adapted adjusted, and distilled from various acknowledged sources but the over all contents and messages are the same. It is the sine qua non for prevention or protection against infections especially in children. That is the essence of immunization.

Essential Family and Travellers' Health

IMMUNISATION SCHEDULE FROM SUMMER 2015

1. AGE	INFECTION PROTECTED AGAINST
AGE	INFECTION IMMUNISED AGAINST
2 Months Old	1. Diphtheria
(First Doses)	2. Tetanus
	3. Pertussis (Whooping Cough)
	4 Polio
	5. Haemophilus Influenza type b (Hib)
	6. Pneumococcal Disease
	7. Meningococcal group B Disease (Men B)
	8. RotaVirus
3 Months Old	1. Diphtheria (Second Dose)
(Note, these are all	2. Tetanus (Second Dose)
Second Doses	3. Pertussis (Second Dose)
Except Meningococcal	4. Polio (Second Dose)
Group C Disease-	5. Haemophilus (Second Dose)
Men C which is	Influenzae type b (Hib)
First Dose	6. Meningoccocal
	Group C Disease (Men C)
	7. Rotavirus (Second Dose)
4 Months	1. Diphtheria
Note these are 3rd	2. Tetanus
Doses but Men B	3. Pertussis
And Pneumococcal	4. Polio
Vaccines are 2nd doses	5. Haemophilus Influenzae b (Hib)
	6. Meningococcal B (Men B)
	7. Pneumococcal Disease
Between 12 and 13	Hi b/Men C

Dr. Usen Ikidde

Months	
	Pneumococcal Disease
	Measles, Mumps, Rubella.(MMR) Live vaccine, 1st Dose
	Meningococcal B - booster though some might not give again
2,3 and 4 years old	Influenza -Flu nasal spray from September-annual
And children in school	
Years 1 and 2	
3 Years 4 months old	Diphtheria
	Tetanus
	Pertussis
	Polio
	Measles, Mumps and Rubella (MMR)
Girls aged 12-13 years	Human Papillomavirus types 16 and 18 (and genital
	Warts caused by types 6 and 11) HPV Gardasil vaccine vaccine.
About 14 years old	1, Tetanus
	2. Diphtheria
	3. Polio
	4 Meningococcal Group C (Men C)
	5. Meningococcal Group W Disease (MenW)5
65 Years Old	Pneumococcal Disease Vaccine (Pneumovax II)
65 Years and Older	Influenza (Flu injection) Annual
70 Years Old	Shingles (Zostavax)
IMMUNISATION FOR THOSE AT RISK	
At Birth, I Month Old, 2 Months Old and 12 Months Old	Hepatitis B
At Birth	BCG Vaccine (Tuberculosis)
6 Months to 2 Years	Influenza (Inactivated Flu Vaccine)

Essential Family and Travellers' Health

2 Years up to Under 65 years of Age	Pneumococcal Disease Vaccine
Above 2 but less than 18 years old	Influenza (Flu Nasal Spray)
13-18 Years Old	Meningococcal Disease (Men W vaccine)
18 and up to 65 years	Influenza (Inactivated Flu Vaccine) Annual
At any Age of Pregnancy	Influenza (Inactivated Flu Vaccine)
From 28 Weeks Of Pregnancy	Pertussis Vaccine

CHAPTER TWO

NON-ROUTINE IMMUNISATION PROGRAMME IN THE UK

IMMUNIZATION IN SPECIAL CIRCUMSTANCES- AT RISK GROUPS

There are other at- risk groups in special circumstances where certain infections or diseases require vaccinations which have to be given due to exposure or occupational diseases where the workers exposed to those diseases have to be protected by immunisation. In some cases, immunisation is given to individuals who travel to areas where certain diseases are more prevalent and protection is required. Protection of such persons also prevents the spread of such infections on the return to their local communities or country.

ANTHRAX

Anthrax immunization is for those who have been in contact with imported infected animals and those who actually handle such animals.

The vaccine is made from the antigen of the organism, Bacillus anthracis. The primary immunisation consists of 4 doses and for those who remain exposed to infected animals, annual immunisation should be given. In addition antibiotics may be given also in confirmed cases of exposure.

BOTULISM

The vaccine is polyvalent in the sense that it is made to neutralise different strains of the toxin produced by Clostridium **botulism** (usually A,B,E)

The vaccine is usually given to individuals who have been exposed to Clostridium botulism and also for the treatment of the condition. Unfortunately many people suffer hypersensitivity reactions to the vaccine and pre treatment checks should therefore be carried out before the actual immunisation is effected.

CHOLERA

Cholera is a bacterial infection of the small intestine by vibrio cholerae. The infection results in large amounts of severe watery diarrhoea which may last for days causing severe dehydration and electrolyte imbalance. The dehydration results in sunken eyes, decreased skin elasticity and wrinkling of the skin of the hand and feet.

Cholera may start a few hours or up to about 5 days from ingestion of infected food or water contaminated by human faeces. Insufficiently cooked sea food is another source of infection.

Cholera is another condition that usually requires the administration of cholera vaccine. The vaccine can be given orally or by injection. The oral form is preferred as the injectable form's effectiveness is open to question and has been discontinued in the UK.

Although there is no specific requirement for immunisation for international travel, cholera vaccination is useful for travellers to endemic parts of the world or where there is a current history of epidemic. Immunisation should preferably be carried out at least one week before travelling to endemic areas.

Cholera vaccination, unfortunately does not convey complete protection. The best protection is for travellers to maintain and pay particular attention to food hygiene, drinking water and personal hygiene.

Children over 6 years and adults are usually given 2 doses separated by an interval of 1-6 weeks and children 2-6 years, 3 doses separated again by interval of 1-6 weeks.

HEPATITIS A

Hepatitis A vaccine is not in routine immunisation but is given to those individuals who are considered to be at risk particularly travellers to high risk areas, intravenous drug users, promiscuous individuals, prostitutes, workers exposed to untreated sewage, people who work with primates, laboratory staff whose jobs bring them into direct contact with the virus, the staff and residents of home for people with severe learning difficulties, patients with haemophilia and related conditions who receive plasma derived clotting factors and patients with chronic liver disease.

Hepatitis A immunisation is also usually considered for patients with chronic liver disease especially those with chronic Hepatitis B or C and in individuals who have had close contact with the virus especially within the same household.

It is recommended that those who have come into contact with the virus during an outbreak, that adults should be given a single dose of the monovalent vaccine and children under 16, a single dose of the combined vaccine. This is considered adequate for rapid protection.

In addition to the above active Hepatitis A vaccine, an intramuscular normal immunoglobulin (passive immunisation) is recommended for those with close contact with confirmed cases of hepatitis A with HIV, chronic liver disease, are over 50 years of age or are immunosuppressed.

Prophylaxis (prevention) Hepatitis A vaccination is not usually required for children under 1 year of age if their carers especially those who change their nappies have been vaccinated.

JAPANESE ENCEPHALITIS

Travellers to the Far East may be at risk in areas where the infection is endemic. Laboratory staffs who are exposed to the virus are also at risk of infection.

Japanese encephalitis vaccine is indicated for such groups of people. It is recommended that 2 doses of the vaccine should be given before the exposure and should be completed at least a week before travelling.

RABIES

Rabies vaccine immunization should be offered to people who are at a high risk of being exposed to rabies virus.

Rabies immunisation should be considered for animal handlers, laboratory staff who handle rabies virus, quarantine staff, veterinary surgeons and nurses and field workers who come into contact with wild animals that are likely to be infected, bat handlers and port officials who come into contact with potentially infected animals.

Immunisation is also usually advisable for visitors to remote parts of the world where there is limited and prompt medical care and those living in "endemic" areas.

Rabies vaccine should also be given to pregnant women in areas with a high risk of exposure, limited medical facilities especially if rabies vaccine is of limited supply or unlikely to be available at all.

Immunisation usually requires 3 doses of rabies vaccine and a booster dose for those still considered to be at high risk of exposure especially laboratory staff who handle rabies virus.

It is recommended that following potential exposure to rabies, that the area be cleaned and washed carefully in running water and then with soapy water as soon as possible following the exposure. The wound should be dressed after application of disinfectant but not sutured immediately as that can lead to adherence of the virus to the nerves.

There are no specific conditions to stop post exposure prophylaxis against rabies; pregnancy is not considered a contraindication. Post exposure prophylaxis should be seriously considered in any country where rabies is enzootic (disease affects animals within the region) even when there is no direct evidence that the attacking animal is "infected".

For someone who has already been fully immunised, and has been exposed or attacked by infected animal,2 doses of rabies vaccine is considered to be sufficient.

SMALL POX

Smallpox has been eradicated and therefore no longer poses any risk to society. However, in laboratory workers where pox viruses are handled, the potential risk of infection remains. To this end, a limited supply of the vaccine is usually made available to workers who handle smallpox virus and have to be vaccinated as a precautionary measure.

TICK-BORNE ENCEPHALITIS

Tick-borne Encephalitis is a viral disease transmitted to humans when bitten by infected ticks The initial symptoms are similar to flu and include a high temperature, tiredness, muscle pain and headache.

The symptoms usually last for about a week or slightly more after which the majority of people make a full recovery. Unfortunately a few people develop more serious symptoms of meningitis(infection of the coverings of the spinal cord and brain) or encephalitis(infection of the brain).It is now tick borne encephalitis and may manifest with symptoms of confusion, disorientation, drowsiness, sensitivity to bright light(photophobia),seizures (fits), paralysis and inability to speak. Patients with these symptoms should seek medical help and be admitted to hospital immediately.

Tick-borne encephalitis could affect travellers returning from rural areas of central, northern and eastern Europe including Russia and some countries in the Far East especially Japan and China.

Ticks live in the woodlands, forest, grassland, marshes and riverside meadows. Infection is transmitted when bitten by an infected tick. The virus is present in the tick's saliva which unfortunately also has an anaesthetic effect which numbs pain and so the bite passes unnoticed.

Tick activity is highest in the spring and early summer but a bite by infected tick can occur at any time of the year.

Although Tick-borne Encephalitis is relatively uncommon in the UK but not so in areas where infected ticks are found and WHO estimates10-12000 cases each year but unreported cases make this estimate merely the tip of the iceberg.

The best prevention is to be vaccinated especially as protection is considered relatively effective.

Despite being vaccinated, travellers and inhabitants should still take precaution in tick-infected areas by wearing long sleeve shirts and trousers tucked into boots or socks, use of effective insect repellent and regular checks of the body for ticks especially where they are more likely to hide from view:

- back of knees,
- the groin,
- armpits,
- behind the ears and hairline.

Tick-borne encephalitis vaccine contains inactivated tick-borne encephalitis virus and is recommended for people working in high risk areas and travellers to those areas.

Three(3) doses of the vaccine are given by intramuscular injection into top of shoulder muscle in adults and side of thigh muscle in children. The second dose is usually given after 1-3 months whilst the third dose is given after a further 5-12 months; 0.5 ml for adults up to 16 years of age and children 0.25 ml.

It is recommended that in the elderly, the immune-compromised and those receiving immune-suppressant medication, antibody concentration should be checked 4 weeks after the second dose.

TYPHOID FEVER

This is a bacterial disease caused by Salmonella typhi and transmitted through eating infected food or drinking water contaminated by urine or faeces of infected people.

Symptoms develop within 1-4 weeks after exposure and range from mild to severe. Typically there is a high fever, diarrhoea or constipation, headache, abdominal pains malaise, rose coloured spots on the chest and enlarged liver or spleen. Only some of these signs and symptoms may be present.

There is a carrier state in which the signs and symptoms only manifest during an acute illness.

Prevention is achievable by meticulous attention to details in regular hand washing especially by food handlers, improvement in sanitation and hygiene and the provision of clean and safe drinking water. Chlorination of water has been reported to reduce infection.

Immunisation should be carried out especially for those who travel to endemic areas such as India and the Indian sub continent. Typhoid Vaccine can prevent 50-70% of cases and is effective for up to 7 years and should be given at least 2 weeks before potential exposure to typhoid infection. Live attenuated Salmonella typhi vaccine is given intramuscularly and oral preparation is also available.

Immunisation should be seriously considered for travellers visiting infected areas of the world especially if visiting local people, interacting, eating and drinking with their hosts.

Vaccination should also be given to laboratory workers who are exposed to the bacteria in the course of their work.

Although humans only are infected, but insects especially flies may carry the bacteria from faeces of infected individuals and transmit through food and water.

Diagnosis is clinical and by laboratory investigations. Clinically, attention should be paid to details of possible source of infection especially travellers who have returned from endemic areas, symptoms and signs above, attention to a high fever which tends to peak in the afternoon and may be as high as 40 degrees C.

Laboratory tests include blood culture and detection of the DNA in blood, stool and bone marrow.

Where the infection is strongly suspected, awaiting the result of laboratory test should not stop starting antibiotics which may be life-saving especially in non- immunised individuals where the disease may spread rapidly and could be fatal.

Complications may arise easily in such individuals and include internal bleeding which may require blood transfusion but often not life threatening. Perforation of the bowel leading to peritonitis(infection of the lining of the abdomen) is a serious complication with high fatality if not recognised early enough and adequately managed surgically.

CHICKEN POX

Is also known as Varicella and is caused by Varicella Zoster virus.It is a contagious infection spread by droplets during coughing and sneezing by infected individuals. It can also be contracted through contact with infected surfaces after the blister has burst onto such surface. The virus is then transferred by touching or contact with the surface.

It is worth noting here that the virus that causes **herpes zoster (shingles)** is the same as Varicella Zoster virus that causes chickenpox. They are therefore the same virus. Someone who suffers from shingles may spread the virus to non-immuned people and result in chicken pox. However the reverse is not the case: spread of chickenpox virus does not result in shingles in the short term.

Spread of the infection may occur one or two days before the emergence of symptoms and the spread is by air-borne droplets through coughing and sneezing. The initial manifestations are usually red itchy rashes which form small blisters that crust and form scabs which eventually drop off. Other symptoms may include headache, fever and tiredness.

The disease may be complicated by bacterial infection of the skin, pneumonia and inflammation of the brain.

The severity and spread of the symptoms and rash vary; some children have only a few spots whilst others have rashes in various stages of development covering the entire surface of the body but more likely to be on the face, ears, scalp, under the arms, belly, chest, legs and arms.

The disease tends to be more severe in adults than in children which often appears as a mild disease.

Typically lesions on the skin show various stages of rash, blister, crusts and scab. This combination is probably the easiest aid in the clinical diagnosis of chickenpox.

The incubation period (time of contact with infected person to the development of rash) is about 10-21 days and the symptoms may only last one to two weeks but this is variable and depends on the severity and possible complications.

People only get chickenpox once which means that **life-long** immunity is **acquired by just one episode of chickenpox infection**.

The most common late complication of chickenpox is herpes zoster(shingles) noted above. The reactivation of chickenpox which had remained dormant in nerve tissue for several years, often since childhood, results in shingles.

Infection during pregnancy may spread through the placenta and result in infection of the fetus. This is worse if the infection occurs in the first 28 weeks of pregnancy and may result in fetal Varicella syndrome also called congenital **Varicella** syndrome which results in varying severity of complications which may include underdeveloped fingers and toes and severe malformations of the bladder and anus. Complications affecting the brain may include encephalitis(inflammation of the brain), microcephaly (small brain), hydrocephaly (fluid in brain) and aplasia (underdeveloped organ e.g the brain).There may be changes to the eye which may include the formation of cataracts.

Treatment of chickenpox in children is mostly symptomatic and should include application of:

- Calamine lotion to relieve the itching.
- Paracetamol for pain and to reduce temperature.
- Ibuprofen may occasionally also be given.
- Antiviral medication, Aciclovir for severe cases especially in adults if started early in the first 24 hours of the appearance of rash and in cases with increased risk of complications.

It is worth emphasising here that aspirin must never be given to children suffering from chickenpox because of possible complication of **Reye's syndrome.**

Reye's syndrome is a severe but rare condition which can cause severe brain and liver damage . Reye's syndrome must be treated promptly to prevent permanent brain injury and death.

The condition mainly affects children and young people under 20 years of age .

The signs and symptoms consists of :

- Drowsiness
- Effortless and persistent vomiting
- Fast breathing
- listlessness (lack of enthusiasm and interest)
- Lack of energy or tiredness
- Fits or seizures

- If the condition is not vigorously treated, it may result in more damage and further complications resulting in:
- Delirium, a severe state of mental confusion.
- Personality changes, including irritability
- Aggressive behaviour
- Hallucinations and
- Coma.

Prevention of chickenpox

Chickenpox should be prevented by adopting the measures mentioned above to prevent contact with known cases during the period of infectivity which usually lasts for about a week. The main problem here is the lack of clear clinical signs before the rash appears when sneezing, coughing and contact at this stage is virtually impossible to prevent and isolate the sufferer as overt symptoms and rash have not yet appeared. Fortunately this period only really lasts for about 1-2 days.

The second period of prevention of contact with infected individual is when the rash is actually evident and this period is much easier to avoid any contacts as the rashes, blisters and crust are apparent.

The second and most important method of prevention is by vaccination. In the UK vaccination against chickenpox is not routine. Immunisation is only given to vulnerable groups which include:

- Seronegative children (lacking immunity against chickenpox virus) over one year of age who come into close contact with individuals with a high risk of chickenpox infection.

- Healthcare workers who are seronegative and come into contact with patients who suffer from chickenpox
- Pregnant women who are susceptible to chickenpox infection and
- People who are susceptible to severe chickenpox infection especially the immuno-deficient and those on immunosuppressive therapy.

Whilst a history of chickenpox infection in childhood would virtually ensure immunity, there are people especially health care workers who are uncertain whether they had childhood infection or immunisation. In such cases, vaccination would be the safe option.

Some healthcare workers may develop sub clinical generalised chickenpox infection following immunization which manifests as rash, and blisters. They should avoid contact with patients until crust formation. Those who develop local rash are usually advised to cover the rash to prevent contact with patients.

Varicella-zoster vaccines are live attenuated vaccines used for vaccination against chickenpox in seronegative individuals. Three main vaccines are available: Varilix, Varivax and Zostavax. The latter is used for immunisation against herpes zoster (shingles).

HERPES ZOOSTER (Shingles)

As a result of chickenpox and shingles virus being one and the same but only different in presentation, it is pertinent here to also delve a little bit more into the clinical features of shingles.

As noted above shingles tend to arise in adults after several years by the reactivation of chickenpox virus which had remained dormant for several years in affected nerves.

Unlike chickenpox which is usually widespread, shingles on the other hand is confined to only one side of the body which may be the nerves of the chest wall, abdomen, face or eye.

An attack of shingles is commonly heralded by pain before the rash appears which as noted above is confined to the nerve on one side of the affected body part. Like chickenpox, rash then appears but confined to the affected nerve which on the chest or abdomen may assume a semicircular appearance in conformity to the nerve root which runs from the back to the front. That is the characteristic appearance but often not the whole length of the nerve root is affected and the semicircular pattern is disrupted and the typical appearance may not be immediately evident.

The lesion, like chickenpox is characterised by a reddish itchy rash but unlike it, may be quite burning and painful. Blisters, crust, scab and pain may be prominent features as noted above.

In some cases before the rash appears, there is an early stage with symptoms in the affected area of:

- burning
- tingling
- numbness
- itchiness

And other symptoms of:

- feeling unwell
- headache and
- fever.

An episode of shingles may actually last for 2-4 weeks and the main symptoms may only be the pain followed by the rash.

Pain is an important and often disturbing feature in shingles and may be in the nature of a localised band which may be dull, burning, constant or intermittent. A sharp stabbing pain may occur from time to time and the affected area of the skin may be tender to touch.

In most people, especially young adults, shingles is not usually serious. However in some people particularly in the elderly, the symptoms may be quite severe and the disease prone to complications. Early medical input and treatment is therefore advised to reduce the severity of the pain and other symptoms.

Pregnancy is an indication to see the family doctor. Those with weakened immune system should also seek medical help early.

YELLOW FEVER

Yellow fever is not included in routine immunisation schedule in the United Kingdom and so only in special circumstances is immunisation considered necessary as will be seen later.

Yellow fever is caused by yellow fever virus spread by the bite of female mosquito especially the Aedes aeypti species. The disease is difficult to distinguish from other febrile illnesses.

Yellow fever only affects humans and other primates, and, of course, the mosquito vector mentioned above. The inoculation period (incubation) is 3-6 days which is the time from the mosquito bite to the development of symptoms.

Symptoms are mild in most cases with fever, chills, fatigue, headache, backache, muscle pain, loss of appetite, nausea and vomiting. In mild cases the symptoms only lasts 3-4 days.

In severe cases there is a toxic phase with recurring fever with jaundice due to liver damage and abdominal pains. Liver damage causes jaundice, hence the name yellow fever. Unfortunately half the patients who enter the toxic phase die within 10-14 days, but the other half recover without significant organ damage.

In such serious cases, bleeding may occur from the mouth, nose and into the gut leading to vomiting of blood. There may also be bleeding into the eyes.

Yellow fever is notoriously difficult to diagnose but should be distinguished from other febrile and haemorrhagic diseases especially severe malaria, viral hepatitis (particularly severe forms of hepatitis B and D), leptospirosis, dengue hemorrhagic fever and other fevers. Although blood tests detect yellow fever antibodies produced due to the infection, in the toxic phase this may be too late to prevent severe disease and complications.

Yellow fever is endemic in many countries in Africa, Central and Latin America with an estimated population of up to 500-900 million people who are at risk of infection by the virus. Imported cases of yellow fever are also reported in counties and regions traditionally free from yellow fever particularly in Asia where the conditions for the propagation of the virus are rife.

The toxic phase may be quite serious and accounts for about 20 -percent of deaths but the overall mortality rate is about 3 per cent though in severe epidemic this may rise to 50 percent.

Surviving infection by yellow fever provides lifelong immunity and so immunisation in such individuals is not required.

Man acquires the infection when bitten by a female Aedes aegypti mosquito and related species. The yellow fever virus is taken up by the mosquito when it bites, sucks and ingests the blood of infected person. The virus reaches the stomach of the mosquito, infects the epithelial cells(lining of the stomach), multiplies and gets to the blood system of the mosquito and migrates to the salivary glands. When the mosquito bites and sucks blood, it injects its saliva into the wound of the victim which gets to the blood stream of the person who becomes infected and in this way the cycle continues.

The diagnosis of yellow fever is mostly clinical by recognising the symptoms and signs and taking a good clinical history of visits or recent return from areas of the world where yellow fever is endemic.

There is no specific treatment of yellow fever; the treatment is therefore symptomatic and supportive particularly the treatment of dehydration, respiratory failure and fever mostly in toxic cases.

Prevention revolves around elimination of the vector(mosquito-Aedes egypti and related species) which may involve stopping the breeding of mosquitoes and preventing being bitten by them. Since the primate is another source of infection and transmission to humans, this additional source of infection should be prevented by isolating them from human habitation.

Vaccination remains the single most important and effective measure of preventing yellow fever. In endemic areas especially in parts of Africa, mass immunization should be the norm. Unfortunately these are often poor countries which can ill-afford such measures. It is estimated that for effective immunisation at least 60-80 % of the population should be vaccinated. Generally, following immunisation, immunity is acquired after about 10 days and travelling to endemic areas is only then permitted.

In the UK, yellow fever vaccination is indicated for those:

- who travel or live in parts of the world where the disease is endemic.
- For laboratory staff who handle the virus or clinical materials which might contain the virus.

It should also be noted that:

- Infants under 6 months of age should not be vaccinated as there is a small risk of encephalitis.
- However children 6-9 months may be vaccinated if there is a high risk of yellow fever which can not be prevented by other means.
- Immunity is believed to be for life but there is some uncertainty and therefore a revaccination after 10 years can be recommended.
- Live yellow fever vaccine should not be given to pregnant women as there is a small and theoretical

risk of fetal infection. Any travel to high risk areas should be avoided during pregnancy. Where such a journey is unavoidable, and the risk to the mother outweighs that to the fetus, then immunisation can be given after explanation to the mother and her acceptance of the small risk involved.

CHAPTER THREE

PASSIVE IMMUNITY

As noted above, passive immunity is unlike active immunity as passive vaccines are not derived from extracts of the organisms but from the plasma or serum of someone who has already had the particular infection or been immunised against it by active immunisation.

Passive immunisation is derived from immunoglobulin of such individuals who having already had the infection or have been actively immunised, now have a rich source of antibodies. This is usually a sterile preparation of concentrated antibodies of pooled human plasma which is rich in antibodies and is called immunoglobulin(immune globulin) "Immune" denotes its immunity status as it is made from a rich source of antibodies and "globulin" is a plasma protein from which it is derived.

Human immunoglobulins are available in two main forms, normal or non-specific immunoglobulin or disease specific immunoglobulin. Normal or non-specific immunoglobulin can therefore be used, as the name implies, for a number of conditions whereas disease specific immunoglobulin is specific for a particular disease only.

Pooled immunoglobulin is from human sources and must therefore be properly tested to ensure that it is infection-free from especially such infections as hepatitis B and C and human immunodeficiency virus (HIV) and any other potential infections.

It is now clear why passive vaccine imparts immediate protection because it doesn't have to produce antibodies in the blood of the recipient as this has already been done in the plasma of the donor. For this reason, the period for the onset of its effectiveness is greatly shortened and so is the period or duration of its potency. It can not therefore stimulate the immune system of the recipient to produce antibodies which would have a longer period of onset and its effectiveness as in active immunisation. The advantage of passive immunization is therefore the fast action in the treatment of infections especially when such infection is life-threatening and would have taken a much longer time to commence its action if active vaccine was given.

It is worth noting also that in many cases one can not make the choice of receiving either the active or passive immunization because this may be disease specific. That means that many infections are treated with active immunisation and others by inactive immunisation because the vaccine available is one or the other and the choice of the vaccine is therefore limited.

Fortunately the alternative of either active or passive vaccine is also available in many infections but the choice of vaccine is usually determined not necessarily by artificial or patient's choice but clinical considerations especially the virulence of the infection and the need for speed or otherwise. It is also worth noting again that where immediate treatment is needed, the answer is passive immunisation but where the protection or prevention is required and there is no active or imminent infection, the answer is active immunisation to stimulate the formation of antibodies to fight infection should such infection arise in the future. Active immunity is therefore preferred as the immunity conferred is likely to be longer lasting and in some cases permanent.

Dr. Usen Ikidde

Immunoglobulin

It is important to restate that immunoglobulins are derived from pooled human plasma of immune individuals who have either been vaccinated against the specific infection or have acquired immunity due to infection.

Immunoglobulin are of 3 main types:

1. Normal Immunoglobulin (non-disease specific immunoglobulin)
2. Disease Specific Immunoglobulin
3. Anti-D (Rh) immunoglobulin

Normal Immunoglobulin is prepared from pooled donations of human plasma usually not less than 1000 donations. It contains antibodies (igG) to the following viruses:

- measles
- mumps
- rubella
- hepatitis A and
- other viruses that are prevalent in the community at the time.

Normal immunoglobulin does not contain antibodies to yellow fever virus and therefore cannot be used to treat this infection.

Live attenuated vaccines (active vaccines) should be given about 3 weeks before or 3 months after the injection of normal immunoglobulin as it may interfere with immune response to active immunisation except in the case of yellow fever which as stated above normal immunoglobulin does not contain yellow fever antibodies and so its use is not limited by giving normal immunoglobulin.

Uses of normal Immunoglobulin

It is given by intramuscular injection for the protection of susceptible contacts against:

- infectious hepatitis (**hepatitis A**)
- measles
- rubella to a lesser degree.

Normal immunoglobulin injection produces immediate protection against these infections and usually lasts for several weeks.

Intravenous immunoglobulin injection is also used as a replacement therapy in several conditions where there is lack of or suppressed immunity and these include children with symptomatic Human immunodeficiency virus (HIV) with recurrent bacterial infections.

Occasionally normal immunoglobulin in replacement therapy can be given intramuscularly or subcutaneously but usually the intravenous preparation route is the preferred option.

Intramuscular normal immunoglobulin is given for the prevention of infection in travellers who come into direct contact with confirmed cases of Hepatitis A infection if they have:

- chronic liver disease
- HIV infection
- are immunosuppressed
- are over 50 years of age.

Normal immunoglobulin is given in such cases as soon as possible within 2 weeks of exposure. Please do note that this is passive immunisation. The active immunisation can be given as above at a different time to prevent interference with immune response but may also be given at the same time in a different site if the need for urgency demands.

MEASLES. Normal immunoglobulin can be given intramuscularly or intravenously in the following circumstances:

- Inadequate immunity in children or adults who come into contact with a known case of measles
- non-immune pregnant women who come into contact with a confirmed case of measles
- infants under 9 months who come into contact with measles or are associated with a local outbreak.

It is worth bearing in mind that active measles vaccine is given routinely in the United Kingdom but the normal immunoglobulin- passive immunisation here is only a further step for some susceptible individuals who come into contact with measles.

Normal immunoglobulin is not effective in the prevention of **rubella.** It is therefore not recommended either for children or pregnant women who have been exposed to rubella. Routine active immunisation with combined vaccine -Mumps, Measles and Rubella (**MMR**) is recommended and is the gold standard in the UK.

Disease Specific Immunoglobulin-

This is usually obtained by pooling the plasma of human donors with high levels of antibodies which is specific to the particular infection required.

Unfortunately there is no specific immunoglobulin for hepatitis A, measles or rubella. As noted above normal immunoglobulin can be used except in rubella in which active immunisation is recommended as in routine immunisation schedule.

Disease specific immunoglobulin is useful in the following infections-

1. Heptitis B
2. Rabies
3. Tetanus
4. Chickenpox

1.HEPATITIS B

Disease specific hepatitis B immunoglobulin is useful when used in combination with active immunisation with Hepatitis B vaccine under the following conditions:

a. prevention of infection in laboratory staff who has been accidentally inoculated with hepatitis B virus
b. other personnel who have been inadvertently injected with hepatitis B virus
c. Infants of mothers who have become infected by Hepatitis B virus during pregnancy
d. Infants of mothers who are hepatitis B carriers and considered high risk of passing the infection to the child

Fortunately hepatitis specific immunoglobulin will not inhibit antibody response when given at the same time with hepatitis B active immunisation. However it is recommended that they should be given at different sites.

2.RABIES

This is another condition in which disease specific immunoglobulin is useful and should be given under the following circumstances:

- where there is exposure of an unimmunised person to an animal that has been brought from a country where the risk of rabies is high. It is also recommended in the country where there is no proper immunisation of animals against rabies and the risk of exposure of human to animals is high.

It is recommended that under those circumstances and the individual has been bitten by such animal, the site of the bite should be washed thoroughly with soapy water and the disease specific immunoglobulin injected directly around the site of the bite or if that is not possible then the thigh should be used.

Rabies vaccine (active immunisation) should also be administered into a different site of the thigh intramuscularly at the same time. This should not be delayed.

3 TETANUS.

Tetanus specific immunoglobulin is useful in tetanus prone wounds. This should be combined with proper cleansing of the wound, appropriate antibiotics and tetanus vaccine. This procedure is also applicable in an established case of tetanus.

Tetanus specific immunoglobulin is given intramuscularly in both the post-exposure prophylaxis and in an established case of tetanus, both in combination with other forms of management above.

4. CHICKEN POX

The varicella -zoster (specific) immunoglobulin(VZIG) is recommended for those people who have no antibodies to the chickenpox virus and are considered to be at a high risk of exposure to chickenpox or herpes zoster (shingles). Those at high risk of infection include:

- women exposed at any stage of pregnancy to chickenpox or shingles. They should be given VZIG within 10 days of exposure.
- newborn babies whose mothers develop chickenpox within a week before or a week after delivery.
- newborn babies considered susceptible to chickenpox who become exposed to the virus in the first week of life.
- Babies in intensive care who are susceptible to the virus and become exposed during the period and
- immunocompromised individuals including those on steroids.

Varicella-zoster immunoglobulin is normally given by intramuscular injection to susceptible individuals not later than 10 days after exposure to chickenpox.

Anti-D (Rh) Immunoglobulin

The main and very important use of Anti-D immunoglobulin is to prevent a rhesus negative mother from forming antibodies against a rhesus positive fetus (baby) she is pregnant with.

This will only occur under the following circumstances:

- The mother is rhesus negative(RhD negative)
- The baby is rhesus positive (RhD positive)
- The mother has previously been exposed to a rhesus positive (RhD positive) blood and therefore developed an immune response against it by sensitisation.

We as humans belong basically to one of 4 blood groups which may be A,B,AB or O. Each of these blood groups may be rhesus positive or rhesus negative. Whether we are rhesus positive or negative is determined by the presence or absence of the rhesus D (RhD)antigen found on the surface of our red blood cells.

When people have this rhesus antigen, they are rhesus positive and those who have none are rhesus negative.

It is estimated that in the UK about 85 per cent of the population are rhesus positive.

Our blood type and genetic factors depend on the genes we inherit from our parents. Whether we are rhesus positive or negative simply depends on how many copies of these rhesus genes (RhD) we have inherited. We may then inherit one from each parent and become rhesus positive, from one parent only and still be rhesus positive but if we don't inherit from either parent at all, then we are rhesus negative.

We can, of course, only inherit the rhesus genes if our parents are themselves rhesus positive and it also depends on whether they have 2 copies or one copy.

It follows that a rhesus negative woman can have a rhesus positive baby if her husband is rhesus positive. If the father has 2 copies of the rhesus antigen gene, all the children will be rhesus positive (as he will give at least one rhesus antigen gene to each child). If, however, the father only has one copy of the rhesus gene then there is only half the chance (50%) of the baby being rhesus positive or negative.

The problem of sensitisation only applies if the mother is rhesus negative and has been previously sensitised to rhesus positive blood. This occurs if the mother is exposed to rhesus positive blood for the first time and the develops an immune response to it.

Immune response is the process whereby the mother's immune system recognises the presence of foreign antigen, the rhesus D factor, and makes antibodies to destroy it.

It is worth noting that the antibodies are usually not manufactured fast enough in the first pregnancy to harm the baby at that stage but in subsequent pregnancies this could easily occur for rhesus negative mother carrying a rhesus positive baby as the antibodies are already present in the mother's blood and waiting to attack the red blood cells of a rhesus positive child in the womb.

Sensitisation occurs under the following circumstances:

1. The rhesus negative mother's blood may be exposed to the baby's rhesus positive blood during delivery.
2. The baby's rhesus positive blood cells may cross into the blood of a rhesus negative mother and it only requires a few blood cells to do so to instigate sensitisation in the mother's blood..
3. There is a good chance of fetal/maternal mixing of blood if there is bleeding during pregnancy.

4. Trauma to the mother's abdomen may cause some mixing of a few blood cells from baby to mother.
5. Carrying out certain invasive procedures such as amniocentesis during pregnancy may also lead to some mixing of blood.
6. Miscarriage and ectopic pregnancy may also lead to some mixing of blood cells to cause sensitisation, antibody production against future rhesus positive babies, haemolysis and jaundice.
7. In the UK, it is rare for a Rhesus negative mother to receive Rhesus positive blood transfusion by mistake but could easily occur in the developing world where medical services may be in their infancy, and is one cause of sensitisation.

Rhesus Disease

When sensitisation has occurred, the next time the woman is exposed to rhesus positive blood, her system would produce antibodies immediately.

If this rhesus negative mother is carrying a rhesus positive baby, the antibodies could lead to a rhesus disease when these antibodies cross the placenta and attack the baby's red blood cells and haemolyse(destroy) them. Haemolysis usually manifests as jaundice in the baby.

Anti-D (Rh) Immunoglobulin

The Anti-D immunoglobulin is obtained and prepared from the plasma of rhesus negative donors who have been immunised against the anti-D antigen.

Anti-D immunoglobulin is used when a rhesus negative mother is pregnant with a rhesus positive baby. It prevents the formation of antibodies against rhesus positive red blood cells which might have passed from the fetal blood to maternal blood. In this way protection is afforded to future pregnancies with rhesus positive fetus(unborn baby) from the hazard of **haemolytic disease of the newborn.**

Haemolytic disease of the new born occurs when the rhesus negative mother's sensitised blood and antibodies cross the placenta to the fetal circulation. When this occurs, there is haemolysis (destruction of red cells) of the rhesus positive fetus. This manifests as jaundice as the liver cannot cope with the removal of the product of the haemolysis(bilirubin) which gives the yellowness of the eyes and skin. The destruction of the red blood cells may also lead to anaemia. In severe cases, there may be other complications such as internal swelling, reduced muscle tone, weakness, poor feeding, and increased breathing.

These symptoms depend on the severity of the condition. In about half of the babies, the symptoms are mild and quite easy to deal with. It is also worth mentioning that haemolytic disease of the new born affects only the baby and the mother won't experience any symptoms or problems.

Anti-D immunoglobulin should be administered to the mother following any of the sensitising episodes enumerated above. It should preferably be administered within 72 hours of such an episode taking place but protection could still be afforded even after this time period has elapsed. The dose of the Anti-D immunoglobulin given should depend on the degree of exposure to the rhesus positive blood.

Routine anti-D immunoglobulin prophylaxis is given when there is none of the sensitising factors above. Under the circumstance, NICE guideline stipulates either 2 doses at

28 and 34 weeks of gestation or one larger dose between 28 and 30 weeks.

Routine anti-D prophylaxis is usually given during antenatal care irrespective of whether a previous dose had been given due to a sensitising episode during the pregnancy.

A postpartum anti-D prophylaxis is also usually given irrespective of routine doses at antenatal or sensitising episode early in the pregnancy.

CHAPTER FOUR

DISEASE PREVENTION IN INTERNATIONAL TRAVEL

International travel poses a significant risk in the exposure of travellers and the spread of diseases. This risk could be minimised or eliminated if adequate prophylactic measures are put in place, prevalence of certain infections in specific geographical areas are recognised and appropriate actions are taken accordingly.

There are several obstacles to this: the increasing porosity of national borders, migration and failure of travellers to recognise and take seriously routine and prophylactic immunisations before embarking on a journey. When these measures are adequately enforced and there is recognition by individuals of their roles in personal safety and the society at large, then much of the problems would have been laid to rest.

There are several infections which international travellers are particularly prone to. Some of these have been dealt with under routine and none routine immunisation schedules and are dealt with here again for emphasis and to highlight other areas of concern. There are others which require preventive measures which may be oral, or injection and non- immunisation measures.

Secondly, I wish to mention as many of these infections as possible but only discuss a few in any degree of details, not because they are unimportant but because there are not widely distributed in large geographical areas and a mere mention would suffice.

On the other hand malaria, for example, is so widely distributed in tropical and a few subtropical areas and travellers are more likely to travel into endemic areas than they would be to some other areas, for example, the West Nile Virus or MERS (Middle East Respiratory Syndrome).This does not, however, diminish the importance or virulence of the latter group of infections.

Secondly since some of these infections have already been described either under routine immunisation or non-routine immunisation they are only included here again for completion and to help travellers identify infections which should be borne in mind during travel. For this reason some of the diseases that have already been described or mentioned are dealt with again under this heading.

Some of the diseases require taking adequate prophylactic (preventive) measures and prompt treatment as there are no vaccines for some of the infections.

Here is a list of most of the infections which travellers should be aware of ant take all necessary precautions before, during and even after a trip:

1. Malaria
2. Tuberculosis (TB)
3. Yellow Fever
4. Hepatitis A
5. Hepatitis B,C,E
6. Typhoid
7. Cholera
8. Diptheria
9. Poliomyelitis
10. Ebola
11. Japanese Encephalitis
12. Tick-borne Encephalitis
13. Lassa Fever

14. Chickenpox
15. Influenza Virus (Flu)
16. Sexually Transmitted Diseases (STD)-Gonorrhoea, HIV, Syphilis, Chlamydia etc (See Chapter Five)
17. Measles
18. African Trypanosomiasis (Sleeping Sickness)
19. Avian Flu (Bird Flu)
20. Dengue
21. Hand, Foot and Mouth Disease
22. Leptospirosis
23. Menincoccocal Disease (Neisseria meningitides)
24. Mumps
25. Murray Valley Encephalitis Virus
26. Pneumococcal Disease (Streptococcus pneumonia)
27. Rabies
28. Rift Valley Fever
29. Rubella
30. Scabies
31. Shistosomiasis
32. Tetanus
33. West Nile Virus
34. MERS (Middle East Respiratory Syndrome)
35. SARS (Severe Acute Respiratory Syndrome)
36. Zika virus

These are some of the most important infections that the traveller might come into contact with. Some are quite common and others far less so. This variation is due to a number of factors: the size of the geographical distribution, the degree of endemicity or prevalence of the virus or infection, susceptibility factors, likelihood of contact and the virulence of the organisms that cause the infections.

1.MALARIA.

Malaria occupies a pivotal and special place amongst the infections which have to be taken very seriously. This is because of the virulence of malaria parasite and the large geographical area in which the vector -female anopheles mosquitoes are found.

Malaria is endemic in tropical and many subtropical regions of the world which stretches from tropical regions of South America, sub-Saharan Africa to tropical and subtropical regions of Asia. Sub-Saharan Africa bears the brunt of this disease with an estimated mortality of about 367000-755000 in 2013 world-wide. Most of the deaths occur in Africa where it is estimated that a child dies every minute with malaria related disease.

Most deaths occur in children who have little or no immunity against the disease. It is estimated that malaria mortality rate has fallen by up to 47% since 2000 worldwide and by 54-58% in African children.

Malaria is transmitted by the female anopheles mosquito which transmits the parasite, Plasmodium, to humans. There are 4 main species of Plasmodium which cause malaria in humans:

1. **Plasmodium falciparum,**
2. **Plasmodium vivax,**
3. **Plasmodium ovalae**
4. **and Plasmodium malariae.**
5. **The 5th species, Plasmodium knowlesi is rare and hardly responsible for any disease in humans .**

Plasmodium falciparum is the most virulent and is responsible for most of the deaths and complications caused by malaria. It is the most likely species to cause infection in travellers especially in the UK and possibly world wide.

Malaria is diagnosed mainly by taking a good clinical history of recent travel to a malarious area of the world, by signs and symptoms and confirmed by microscopic examination of blood film or by antigen based rapid diagnostic tests.

The symptoms of malaria may include non- specific symptoms of:

- Fever
- Headache
- Vomiting
- Tiredness
- Sweating with chills
- Diarrhoea
- Cough
- Muscle pain and
- Tenderness.
- Major clinical features of complications due to falciparum malaria in children may include any of the following:
- Seizures
- Impaired consciousness
- Breathing difficulties
- Acidosis (blood becomes more acidic than normal)
- Low blood sugar (hypoglycaemia)
- Anaemia which may be severe
- Severe weakness and inability to stand
- Major clinical features of complication of falciparum malaria in adults include:

- Fits or seizures
- Low blood Sugar
- Anaemia
- Acute respiratory Syndrome
- Pulmonary Oedema
- Disseminated Intravascular Coagulation(clotting of blood within the circulation)
- Bleeding
- Haemoglobin in urine
- Shock.
- In severe cases of falciparum malaria, there may be:
- Seizures
- Coma
- and death from cerebral malaria.

The symptoms typically start about 10-15 days after a bite by a female anopheles mosquito. The likelihood of developing symptoms is determined by:

- the number of bites,
- The lack/degree of partial immunity of the individual to malaria
- the species of Plasmodium
- and the general health of the victim may be an additional factor.

An individual who has been bitten by several mosquitoes is more likely to develop the symptoms of malaria. In short, the likelihood of infection is due to the degree of parasitemia (number of parasites in the blood). The more the number, the more the likelihood of developing severe disease and possible complications.

There is no absolute immunity to malaria; individuals who live in endemic areas develop a partial immunity which makes symptoms less severe and in some cases none at all.

It is very important to point out that people from endemic areas who migrate or live abroad lose their partial immunity within months or a few years. In visiting their home country, they require the same stringent prophylactic measures as foreign travellers to that country.

Another important factor in the development of disease is the species of Plasmodium which the individual has been exposed to . As noted above, Plasmodium falciparum is the most dangerous and the transmission by this species is more likely to cause severe disease and lead to the development of complications especially in children and the non-immune.

Susceptibility to malaria infection is worse in the malnourished, people with lowered immunity and the very young infants in endemic areas who have virtually no immunity at all to the parasite.

Let me delve very briefly into the life history of malaria and how it becomes transmitted to affect humans.

When one is bitten by an infected female anopheles mosquito, it injects the parasites into human blood. They are called **sporozoites** at this stage, and there may be a fair number. These then travel to the liver and develop in 5-7 days (Plasmodium falciparum) into **a schizont** with thousands of offspring called **merozoites** which are released into the blood stream when the schizont ruptures. The merozoite has the ability to infect a red blood cell. Once in the red blood cell, the malaria parasite begins to grow and divide and after about 48 hours (P.falciparum, vivax or ovale) or 72 hours

(P.malariae) to form 8-32 parasites.The red blood cells then burst and release them to infect other red blood cells.

As this process continues, the number of infected red blood cells increase and the symptoms of illness manifest.

Usually there are some parasites in the red blood cells that do not divide but instead form sexual stages called **gametocytes**. When a female anopheles mosquito sucks blood from the infected individual, the gametocytes are taken up and mate to complete the malaria cycle.

Antimalarial and preventive measures are targeted at different points in the cycle as follows:

1. bite prevention,
2. developmental stage in the liver and
3. during multiplication of parasites in the red blood cells which is the stage of manifestation of clinical illness.

We shall come to these stages and the preventive measures in a little more detail later under prevention.

It is worth mentioning here that Plasmodium vivax and ovale also have a dormant stage in the liver called **hypnozoites.** As the name suggests, the parasites appear hypnotized at that stage: they are inactive. That stage could last for several months. When they come out of this "hypnotized" stage, they become normal schizonts. **The importance of this stage of dormancy is the fact that a traveller could develop clinical signs of malaria 3-12 months after a return from endemic area making diagnosis difficult unless a good history of having travelled abroad several months back, is taken and due consideration given to the possibility of fever being due to malaria** . A blood film microscopic examination should then be carried out.

It is not unusual for other febrile infection(s) to coexist with malaria and that possibility should also be borne in mind especially when the symptoms are atypical and unresponsive to conventional medical treatment.

If a traveller has received normal and full treatment to get rid of the hypnozoites in the liver,and has not been re-exposed to malaria, then it is unlikely that recurrent or prolonged periods of fever over several months or years is due to malaria.

Prevention

Prevention is the most important part of this discussion because without it after having been to an endemic area, dire consequences could follow. Prevention is divided into different parts which should be combined to ensure effectiveness. These are as follows:

1. Awareness of risk-

Travellers should study the area of the world they intend to travel to, and the possibility of endemicity of malaria, the pattern of drug resistance, the type and virulence of malaria species and the anti malarial medications in use during the time. The family doctor may already know these facts but a traveller's input may also be crucial as sometimes the variables and trend alter rapidly.

2.Prevention of breeding of mosquitoes

This involves the prevention of breeding places and applies more to the residents of endemic regions of the world where malaria is prevalent, than to travellers who visit those regions and have little or no input in stopping the breeding of mosquitoes.

Briefly, the life cycles of mosquitoes take place in standing pools of water, water in cans, pots or containers left outside where rain water collects. In cities, open drains and gutters provide excellent breeding grounds for mosquitoes. It is important to remove, destroy or make it impossible to leave any forms of standing or stagnant water. By so doing the breeding of mosquitoes is prevented at source.

3. Prevention of mosquito bite:

(a)

- Avoid exposure to mosquito by staying indoors especially during dusk and dawn when mosquitoes are more likely to seek a blood meal.
- Wear protective clothing-long sleeve shirt, long trousers and socks.
- Use mosquito Repellent cream.

Repellent cream containing diethyl toluamide (DEET) is the most effective form of bite-prevention.

Insect repellant containing 30-50% of DEET will effectively repel mosquito when applied to exposed skin.

(b) Mosquito nets

It is important for travellers and people living in endemic areas to use insecticide-treated mosquito nets especially if the windows are not fitted with gauze meshing. The net should be small-meshed with no holes which are often caused by damage or rough handling of the net.

Using a mosquito net is unlikely to stop the entry of mosquitoes unless, particular attention is paid to details. One important aspect of this is to ensure that the net is tucked in under the bottom sheet. It should then be rolled up to prevent mosquitoes from gaining entry.

The mosquito net should be treated with insecticide which provides additional measure of protection against mosquitoes.

If you are visiting an endemic area, it is better to buy and travel with your own net than depend on local retailers as the quality of the net could be an important issue which determines the effectiveness of protection against the entry of mosquitoes into the net.

The effect of impregnation of the net usually lasts about 6-12 months on average use. The net should not be washed after re-impregnation with insecticide to ensure potency and effectiveness of protection.

4.Preventive (prophylactic) Medicines .

This is the most important aspect of prevention for travellers but not to inhabitants of endemic regions. Many travellers unfortunately pay little attention to the other measures above and perhaps rightly assume that by sticking to prophylactic medication they could usually achieve about the same result. This is almost true but this writer is of the opinion that a combination of the other measures with medication is the gold standard in the prevention of malaria.

It is important to emphasize again that the preventive medication depends on the region to be visited by the traveller and this in turn depends on the P.falciparum resistance to chloroquine at that particular time.

Dr. Usen Ikidde

Public Health England Advisory Committee on malaria prevention (ACMP) updates it guidelines for malaria prevention for travellers from the UK based on effectiveness, resistance to chloroquine, prevalence of malaria and individual circumstances.

The geographical spread of the resistance to chloroquine and some other drugs have been increasing .It covers sub-Saharan Africa, South East Asia, Indian Subcontinent and some parts of South America.

In general the following medications used singly or in combination are currently in use **and depend on the geographical area of the world to be visited by the traveller:**

1.DOXYCYCLINE AND MALARONE.

(**Malarone** is a combination of Proguanil and Atovaquone)

These are used in areas with chloroquine resistance. Long term use of Malarone requires specialist advice . Malarone should be taken daily and started a day or two before travel and continued for a week after leaving the endemic area.

It is recommended that because of the risk of poor absorption, it should be taken with a meal rich in fat to aid the process of absorption in combination.

Doxycycline is taken daily and should be started a day or two before the travel . It should then be continued for a further 4 weeks on return from the journey.

2 MEFLOQUINE . Is the alternative to Doxycycline or Malarone and like them, it is recommended for chloroquine resistant malaria especially in Africa and other areas of the world with the same problem.

It is not suitable for some people with mental health problems as it may cause mood changes and paranoia.

3. CHLOROQUINE AND PROGUANIL COMBINATION(C+P) is taken weekly and recommended for the few areas without chloroquine resistance. In such areas chloroquine is taken weekly and solely without **proguanil.**

The combination is used in areas with a slightly higher risk of **chloroquine** resistant malaria. Unfortunately because of the shrinking geographical area without chloroquine resistance, the combination has become less effective and is being gradually abandoned.

Proguanil (Paludrine) is taken daily in combination with chloroquine which is taken weekly. Proguanil itself has seen the decline in its effectiveness due to resistant strains of malaria parasite.

The combination is still taken in some parts of the Indian Subcontinent and some other parts of the world considered low risk.

Both drugs should be commenced at least a week before travel and continued for 4 weeks after return from the malarious area.

The combination is not recommended for Africa where chloroquine resistance has posed serious impediments to the use of such medication.

Chloroquine and proguanil are the only anti- malarial prophylactic medication that can be bought without prescription; others usually require your family doctor or pharmacist to authorize their use.

Despite all the preventive measures, there is still a very small risk of the development of malaria infection and possibly causing death if both the patient and doctor are not aware of the full history of travel and more importantly that the disease may still occur even after a year of travel due to the hepatic phase of the parasite explained above.

It is therefore important to keep this in mind if you or a family member who had travelled abroad in the preceding year developed a fever or flu- like illness. Under the circumstances above, it is important to seek medical help as soon as possible and remember to tell the doctor about your itinerary, when you undertook the trip, the preventive measures you took and the symptoms you are experiencing.

Having read this book, it is also vital for you to point out the possibility of malaria to your doctor and not assume that the doctor knows everything because doctors do not know everything; they are only human and many have good medical knowledge and Tropical Medicine is a specialty and not all doctors have had adequate exposure. The author recalls how many doctors used to ask him to handle such cases as they were not comfortable with them.

2.TUBERCULOSIS(TB)

This is a serious bacterial infection spread by inhalation of tiny droplets from the sneeze or cough of an infected person. TB is characterised by persistent cough which usually lasts for more than 3 weeks accompanied by phlegm or sputum which may be blood stained.

There may also be any of the following:

- Night sweats
- Weight loss
- Fever
- Loss of appetite
- Fatigue or persistent tiredness.
- There may be swelling of lymph nodes particularly in the neck.

TB is caused by acid fast bacilli bacterial organism which typically affects the lungs but may also affect other body organs and systems especially the gastrointestinal tract.

Spread is due to or by:

1. Prolonged exposure to infected individual especially within the same family or health care workers who regularly attend to patients who might be unaware of their illness. This close contact makes them more prone to tuberculosis infection.
   Immunised or healthy individuals may be able to resist the infection because of having been immunised or due to the body's natural defence against infection.
2. In a weakened immune system the TB bacteria (Mycobacterium tuberculosis) will spread within the lungs and possibly to other parts of the body and symptoms develop due to active infection.
3. A poorly ventilated room
4. People already weakened by other illnesses
5. Malnutrition and
6. Overcrowding are other factors that aid the spread and susceptibility of individuals to infection.

Dr. Usen Ikidde

Active TB became less common in the UK but there has been a resurgence in the last 20 years especially amongst the immigrant and ethnic minority communities where TB is still endemic in their countries of origin.

In 2013 there were about 8000 cases of TB reported in the UK; about 5000 of those affected were born outside the UK which points to spread within family circles and imported infection during visits to countries of origin where TB is still prevalent. The Indian subcontinent appears to bear the brunt of TB endemicity.

Fortunately TB can be cured though drug resistance is a problem. A six months course of antibiotics is sufficient in most cases. As a result of resistance, a combination of antibiotics is usually the preferred option. Treatment can take as long as 2 years in drug resistant cases.

It is estimated that about a third of people infected globally with latent TB, about a tenth of these will become active at some stage.

People who experience symptoms of TB should see their family doctor without delay as early diagnosis and prompt treatment will help to ensure the possible prevention and spread to others especially within the family and community.

A good history followed by a chest X-ray, blood tests and Mantoux skin test should suffice to make the initial diagnosis and commencement of treatment.

The clinical history should include symptoms, signs, family history of TB, immunisation history and history of trips abroad to countries where TB is prevalent.

TB is particularly prevalent in the following countries and regions of the world:

- South East Asia including India, Pakistan, Indonesia and Bangladesh
- Africa especially Sub-Saharan Africa
- Some parts of Russia
- Parts of China
- South America
- Cambodia
- Vietnam

In fact, no country is entirely exempt due to imported infection from other parts of the world. The speed and convenience of air travel has turned the world into one big "global village" where infection can no longer be contained and confined to political and geographical borders.

It is therefore important that people from any part of the world who experience the above symptoms, even if there had been no known contacts, should not hesitate to see their family doctor. There are advantages and disadvantages of "globalization." This is one of the few disadvantages.

TB is treated by a combination of suitable antibiotics in which the organisms are susceptible in order to overcome the problem of resistance which has become a major problem that is not only confined to TB but to a number of other bacteria including the MRSA(Methicillin Resistant Staphylococcus aureus).Resistance of many organisms to current antibiotics has become a global problem that can no longer be ignored.

Prevention.

Dr. Usen Ikidde

Prevention is a major aspect of the control of spread of TB infection and consists of 2 main prongs of attack:

1. Early recognition of symptoms and treatment to prevent the spread to others especially within the family and community.
2. BCG vaccination which provides effective protection to 80 percent of those vaccinated. Unfortunately BCG vaccination is not included in routine immunisation programme to everyone in the UK. Susceptible age groups, communities and individuals are however able to avail themselves of the opportunity to have BCG vaccination. In particular the newborn from susceptible communities are usually given BCG vaccination especially those with a positive family history of tuberculosis. Parents are therefore encouraged to inform their family doctors to effect vaccination.

Health care workers who are more likely to come into contact with infected patients and young people under 16 who live and work in communities with high rate of infection are also usually given priority in BCG vaccination and should be encouraged to avail themselves of such opportunity.

3.YELLOW FEVER

See above under non- routine immunisation in the UK The relevance for travellers is also articulated there.

EBOLA

Ebola virus disease is an haemorrhagic fever that affects humans and other primates and is caused by the Ebola virus.

The incubation period (time between contact with infected person and development of symptoms) is about 2-21 days.

The **symptoms** are:

Influenza-like illness of:

1. fever
2. muscle and joint pains
3. tiredness
4. weakness
5. poor appetite
6. sore throat

These are followed by a period of:

7. vomiting
8. diarrhoea
9. abdominal pains
10. chest pains
11. shortness of breath
12. skin rash
13. internal and external bleeding from the nose, eyes, intestine or skin.
14. In the final stages there are symptoms and signs of impairment of liver and kidney functions.

Death is usually due to hypotension (low blood pressure) occasioned by fluid loss and organ impairment. This could take up to 2 weeks from symptomatic disease.

Dr. Usen Ikidde

Spread is by contact with body fluids especially:

1. blood
2. faeces
3. vomit
4. Semen may carry the virus for several months after recovery from Ebola and so unprotected sexual intercourse is a potential source of infection.
5. saliva
6. urine
7. breast milk may carry the virus for several months after recovery and suckling by a baby may transmit the virus.
8. items recently contaminated by body fluid of infected person.

Also:

Fruit bats are important carriers of infection but themselves show no symptoms of disease.

9. In some African countries where the consumption of bush meat is regarded as the norm, a delicacy and an important source of protein, Ebola virus can easily be contracted either due to the consumption or the handling of infected meat.

Differential diagnosis. It is important to distinguish Ebola from other febrile and haemorrhagic illnesses and infections. These include:

1. malaria
2. typhoid fever
3. cholera
4. meningitis.

Diagnosis is made by history of:

1. a visit to an endemic area and in the last West African outbreak-Guinea, Liberia or Sierra Leone.
2. inadvertent contact with body fluid of an infected person
3. history of contact with animals in the area
4. signs and symptoms of Ebola above
5. Blood samples which are tested for viral RNA, viral antibodies or identification of the virus itself.

Control of outbreak of Ebola.

Ebola outbreak can be controlled by the following methods:

1. Co ordination of medical services and community involvement in the control
2. Detection of infected persons
3. Contact tracing
4. Isolation of infected individuals
5. Proper handling of body fluids of infected people
6. Limitation and prevention of spread of disease from infected animals to humans
7. Wearing of protective gloves, clothing , boots , gowns whilst handling infected body fluids, infected individuals, and any surgical instruments used in the management of the patients should be properly disposed of.
8. Proper washing of hands
9. Education of the community against the traditional hunting, slaughter and eating of bush meat.
10. The use of non -specific vaccine which is now available
11. The use of a new vaccine, Zmapp, is in experimental stage and not yet fully tested in humans. Its use has not been discouraged in

desperate cases and has so far been reported to have shown positive results.
12. Supportive treatment should include oral hydration therapy, intravenous fluid for those unable to tolerate oral hydration which may be due to excessive vomiting or those who require immediate and large quantity of fluids.
13. All travel to infected regions should be discouraged except for health care workers who are well equipped and wear protective clothing, gloves, masks and boots to prevent any contact with infected body fluids and materials. Visits to infected countries during epidemic should only be undertaken if absolutely necessary except for medical personnel and other field workers.

Regional outbreak and a brief history of Ebola

The last outbreak occurred in West Africa and three countries bore the full brunt of the epidemic. These were Guinea, Sierra Leone and Liberia and the infection is thought to be now virtually eradicated.

The first known Ebola outbreak was in the Congo in 1976 near the Ebola river from which the disease derives its name. Since then, there had been intermittent outbreaks in Tropical Africa but the worst was the recent outbreak in West Africa which 10-12 thousand people died.

A total of 24 outbreaks have been reported by the World Health Organisation (WHO) between 1976 and 2013.

LASSA FEVER

It is not inconceivable for travellers to come into contact with Lassa fever despite the restricted geographical location in West Africa especially in the following countries:

- Sierra Leone,
- Guinea,
- Nigeria and
- Central African Republic.

It is, however, very likely that the neighbouring countries are equally affected but no proper studies or investigations have been carried out.

Lassa fever is an acute viral illness which may lead to bleeding .It was first discovered and described in Northern Nigeria in 1969 in a town called Lassa when two missionary nurses died from the disease. This haemorrhagic disease is therefore named after the town, Lassa, where the first cases occurred..

The virus is animal-borne (zoonotic). It is a single-stranded RNA virus and a member of the family Arenaviridae which resembles the Ebola virus though slightly different modes of transmission.

The virulence, infectivity and the clinical features of Lassa fever are slightly milder than Ebola. This may explain but not justify why it has received less publicity, funding, attention and its exclusion from WHO list of neglected tropical diseases which would have raised its profile and recognition as a deadly disease. Such inclusion would help to mobilize opinion as well as national and international resources to help in its management and eradication.

Dr. Usen Ikidde

There is currently an outbreak in Nigeria in 2016 and so far unspecified number of people have died. Actual morbidity and mortality figures are not yet available but health authorities are doing everything possible to limit the infection and reduce individual and geographical spread. The lack of any border control in the ECOWAS sub region means that the neighbouring countries are also very likely to be affected and any of them might have been the source of unreported initial outbreak of this infection.

Transmission

A. The animal host is a rodent- mouse or multimmamate rat (Mastomys natalensis) which harbours the virus in faeces or urine and transmits the virus to susceptible individuals who come into contact with infected urine or faeces of the rodent. The animals frequent grain stores in residences and this is a likely source of contact.
B. Unfortunately transmission also occurs through droplets or inhalation of tiny particles of infected material.
C. through skin injury and
D. worst still transmission also occurs from person to person through close contact with infected material, presenting a risk to travellers and healthcare workers.
E. There is also the very likelihood of transmission by sexual contact.
F. Like Ebola, there is no evidence of airborne person to person transmission. This should be distinguished from transmission through the inhalation of infected rodent's material stated above and person to person transmission through infected material stated in (D)

In West Africa Lassa fever affects 300,000-500,000 people annually and results in about 5000 deaths each year. Though not universally known and recognised as an important cause of ill heath and death, given the high incidence rate, prevalence, morbidity and mortality, it is a major health problem in affected areas.

In about 80% of cases, the disease is asymptomatic but in the remainder, complications could follow. The incubation period is about a week to three weeks and may involve many organs with non specific symptoms of:

- Fever
- Muscle pains and fatigue,
- Swelling of the face,
- Mucosal bleeding and
- Conjunctivitis.
- Other organs may be involved as follows:
- Respiratory tract
- Cough
- Shortness of breath
- Chest pain
- Pleuritis
- Pharyngitis.
- Cardiovascular System
- Hypertension
- Hypotension
- Tachycardia (fast heart rate)
- Pericarditis
- Gastro intestinal tract
- Nausea
- Vomiting which may contain blood
- Diarrhoea possibly with blood in the stool
- Constipation
- Stomach ache
- Difficulty in swallowing (dysphagia)

- Inflammation of the liver (hepatitis)
- The central nervous system may be affected by:
- Meningitis
- Encephalitis
- Fits and
- Partial deafness which may involve one or both ears.

Prevention and Treatment of Lassa fever

1. The control of the rodent (Mastomys) population is by keeping them away from homes and food supplies. Some communities use mousetrap and pesticides and find them useful.
2. Avoidance of contact with the rodent and any waste materials left by them.
3. The rodents particularly target grains as their main item of food and storage of such food items at home should be avoided. Barns can be used and adequate measures adopted to keep out the rodents.
4. Effective personal hygiene which should include regular washing of hands if there is any suspicion of contact with the rodents or their waste material.
5. The use of laboratory coats, masks, gloves and goggles should be encouraged if there is the possibility of contact with infected person.
6. Research is ongoing for the production of effective vaccine especially at the USAMRIID facility by military biologists who study infectious diseases.
7. There should be proper isolation of infected persons; their body fluids and waste products should be disposed of properly.
8. Ribavirin is a drug (a prodrug) that interferes with viral replication by inhibiting RNA-dependent nucleic acid synthesis. This drug has shown an initial success and effectiveness especially when given intravenously rather than orally.

9. Patients should have effective rehydration, blood transfusion and measures taken to combat hypotension.
10. The use of intravenous interferon may prove useful.
11. Induction of labour in the third trimester is necessary if the mother is to have a good chance of survival because the virus has a high affinity for highly vascular tissues such as the placenta.Unfortunately the fetus has a minimal chance of survival, in the order of 10% and hence the emphasis should be on the mother. After induction the mother should receive the same level of care as other infected patients.
12. Analysis of prognosis shows about 15-20% mortality in hospitalised patients with an overall mortality rate of 1%, but during epidemic, mortality could be as high as 50%. In the first trimester of pregnancy, maternal mortality could be as high as 80% with virtually no chance of fetal survival.
13. Pregnant women should be advised to avoid visiting infected regions during LASSA fever epidemic; fortunately this is rare.

MEASLES

Measles is included in routine immunization in the UK and many other countries. Unfortunately there are still a few countries in the developing world where there are no adequate provisions for routine immunization.

It is a highly infectious viral illness which is common in young children and can result in serious complications.

Travellers with children to those countries where measles is still prevalent should ensure that their children are adequately vaccinated before they make such trips abroad.

Dr. Usen Ikidde

Despite being far more common in children, anyone who has never been vaccinated can still get measles.

The symptoms of measles develop about 10 days after exposure before the appearance the typical skin rash.

Symptoms include:

1. Red sore eyes
2. Cold -like symptoms, sneezing, runny nose and cough
3. A high temperature of 38-40 degrees C.
4. Careful examination reveals small greyish-white spots on the inside of the cheeks or under the tongue (Koplik's spots).Not every child would have these spots and so absence does not exclude measles.
5. Loss of appetite
6. Aches and pains
7. Irritability
8. Tiredness and lack of energy.

Spread

Measles is an airborne disease which spreads via droplets especially through coughing and sneezing by infected people. Saliva and nasal secretions are also other avenues of spread. Infection is spread to others by breathing of the droplets or when sneezing or coughing onto surfaces and other people become exposed to the droplets, though the virus can survive there for a few hours only, after which there is no risk of infection.

Infectivity begins from the appearance of symptoms to about 4 days after the appearance of the rash.

The Rash

Measles rash is typically red and flat. It tends to start on the face and spread to the trunk and limbs usually in about 3-5 days after the beginning of symptoms which could last for a week to 10 days.

Complications.

Complications make measles a serious infectious disease and may include any of the following:

1. Severe diarrhoea
2. vomiting
3. Dehydration
4. Conjunctivitis (eye infection)
5. Otitis media (ear infection)
6. Laryngitis
7. Inflammation of the brain(encephalitis)
8. Blindness
9. Pneumonia
10. Bronchitis
11. Croup
12. Meningitis
13. Febrile convulsions
14. Hepatitis (inflammation of the liver)
15. Miscarriage or still birth in pregnant women
16. Prematurity
17. Low birth weight
18. Chest complications may cause shortness of breath requiring emergency care.
19. Shortness of breath and/or sharp chest pain
20. Brain complications may cause drowsiness, confusion and seizures which may require emergency care.

Only about 1 in 15 of children will develop complications which are more likely to occur in children with:

1. weakened immune system,
2. malnutrition or poor diet,
3. leukaemia,
4. children less than a year old,
5. Also teenagers and adults tend to have more cases of complications.

Prevention

In the UK measles is included in routine immunization programme by having the MMR vaccine (measles, mumps and rubella). The first dose is given between 12-13 months of age and the second dose at about 3 years 4 months of age. See current immunization schedule in chapter one.

Older children and adults can have the vaccine at any age if they have not been fully vaccinated before.

In special circumstances MMR can be given to children over 6 months of age or adults if there is immediate risk of infection as follows:

1. Travelling abroad to parts of the world where infection is rife
2. You recognize that you have come into close contact with infected person.
3. There is an outbreak of measles in your area of residence.

In younger children, they would still need to have the routine immunisation at the appropriate age despite having had the vaccine in any of the special circumstances above.

Essential Family and Travellers' Health

Human Immunoglobulin (passive immunity) should also be given to people under special circumstances already alluded to above but in particular:

1. Pregnant women with no clear history of previous immunisation and who have not had measles infection before.
2. Individuals with weak immune system
3. This includes those with HIV
4. Leukaemia cases undergoing treatment
5. Babies under 6 months of age who have been exposed to someone with measles.

Prevention should also include:

1. avoidance of contact with someone who has measles
2. If your child has measles, he/she should not attend school in the first 4 days of the appearance of measles rash.
3. Avoidance of contact should be observed with others especially those who are more likely to be badly affected such as young children and pregnant women.

Treatment.

The treatment of measles is symptomatic; there is no specific treatment. However, you should avoid contact with others in the first 4 days of appearance of the rash.

The following measures may prove useful:

1. Take Paracetamol or Ibuprofen to bring down high temperature and relieve the aches and pains.

2. It is advisable to take plenty of fluids if there is risk of dehydration especially in the face of vomiting or diarrhoea.
3. Conjunctivitis is best treated with chloramphenicol eye ointment which your doctor can prescribe for you or your child.
4. Patients with complications are particularly advised to see their doctor or attend the nearest Accident and Emergency Department and see a doctor who under certain circumstances would refer them to appropriate specialist.

AFRICAN TRYPANOSOMIASIS (SLEEPING SICKNESS)

African Trypanosomiasis (or sleeping sickness) occurs in 36 sub-Saharan African countries. It is endemic in these countries and therefore not inconceivable that travellers to Africa, especially those who visit and spend some time in the rural areas, could come into contact with this disease.

The disease is caused by a flagellate protozoan **Trypanosoma brucei** and is transmitted to human hosts by the bites of **tsetse fly.**

There are 2 types of Trypanosoma brucei that infect humans,**Trypanosoma brucei gambiense** and **Trypanosoma brucei rhodesiense.**

The vast majority(over 98%) of African Trypanosomiasis are caused by Trypanosoma brucei gambiense.

After about 1-3 weeks of a bite by an infected tsetse fly, the following symptoms and signs could occur:

1. Intermittent fever
2. Joint pains

3. Headache
4. Itchiness
5. Marked lymphadenopathy (swelling of lymph nodes)
6. Red sore at the site of bites by tsetse fly may be apparent.
7. If unrecognised and left untreated there may be anaemia, heart, kidney and endocrine dysfunctions.

The second stage begins after several weeks or months with neurological phase of the disease when the parasite invades the central nervous system after passing through the blood-brain barrier and the disturbance of sleep cycle is the main symptom at this stage. The name, sleeping sickness, is derived from this disruption which causes sleep disturbances especially daytime drowsiness and sleepiness. There may be:

1. Confusion
2. numbness
3. Poor coordination
4. Problem getting to sleep at night
5. Irregular, disorganised and fragmented 24 hour rhythm of sleep.
6. Excessive sleep during the day
7. Night time wakefulness (insomnia)
8. General muscle weakness
9. Hemiparesis and paralysis of a limb may occur.
10. Tremor
11. Psychiatric symptoms may include:
12. Aggressive behaviour
13. Irritability
14. Apathy
15. Psychosis

Armed with possible evidence of having been to endemic area and manifestation of early symptoms, the next course of action is to confirm the diagnosis immediately without waiting for deterioration to neurological disease by:

1. Blood smear to find the parasite
2. Possibly also in the fluid of a lymph node
3. Lumbar puncture may be necessary to differentiate the first from second stage disease.
4. It is also possible to obtain fluid by aspiration of fluid from skin of bite site and subject to microscopy for presence of the parasite.

The disease becomes invariably fatal with development of neurological symptoms unless treatment is instituted early. There is progressive mental deterioration, systemic organ failure, coma and death.

Untreated infection by Trypanosoma brucei gambiese will cause death if untreated after several years whereas T.b. rhodesiense disease causes death within months.

Trypanosoma brucei rhodesiense infection despite being far less common

(less than 2% of cases) is far more serious and deadly than trypanosoma gambiense.

Prevention

There is no available vaccine for this disease.

Prevention options include the following:

1. Tsetse fly insect repellents
2. Avoidance of tsetse fly infested areas
3. Wearing long trousers, socks, boots and long sleeve shirts to prevent tsetse fly bites

4. Bush clearing to prevent tsetse fly habitat
5. Wild game culling
6. Systemic screening of at risk communities is sine qua non if this disease is to be eradicated.
7. Active detection and prompt treatment of new infections is imperative.
8. A systematic active surveillance should be adopted.

The measures above should have a multi agency participation or organisational approach involving the World Health Organization (WHO), African Union, individual African countries, charities, Public Health Departments, international institutions and governments concerned and dedicated to the eradication of this deadly disease.

At the 25th International Scientific Council for Trypanosomiasis Research and Control (ISCTRC) in Mombasa, Kenya in October 1999, an African initiative to control the insect vector-tsetse fly and Trypanosomiasis were discussed.

The African Union meeting at its 36th summit in Lome, Togo in July 2000 passed a resolution to form the Pan African Tsetse and Trypanosomiasis Eradication Campaign (PATTEC). The main thrust of this initiative was the campaign to eradicate or reduce the tsetse fly population, consequently and subsequently Trypanosomiasis by the widespread use of insecticide targeted at the vector population, use of fly traps, ultra-low dose aerial/ ground spraying of tsetse fly resting sites(SAT), the use of sterile insect technique

(SIT) and insecticide-treated cattle.

The use of sterile insect technique (SIT) was adopted in Zanzibar, a small island, off the coast of East Africa. SIT involves the release of overwhelming number of sterile insects into the wild. This method proved effective in eliminating tsetse fly from the island. Such method would be impracticable in many African countries with large expanse of land and forest areas which extend beyond national boundaries.

Treatment

Treatment depends on the stage of this disease and can be summarised as follows:

First stage

2. Pentamidine given intravenously or intramuscularly for Trypanosoma brusei gambiense
3. Suramin given intravenously for T.b rhodesiense

Second stage disease

1. Eflornithine given intravenously for T.b. gambiense

Or

1. In combination with Nifurtimox
2. Melarsoprol is now gradually being abandoned in favour of 1 or 2 above. It is still possibly the only treatment available for the neurological phase of T.b.rhodesiense.

It is toxic and causes death in about 5% of people.

Distribution, morbidity and mortality

Sleeping sickness is a major cause of morbidity and mortality in the African continent. The population at risk is estimated to be nearly 70 million people. It is still endemic in South East Uganda and western Kenya and sporadically occur in most of sub-Saharan Africa.

The disease killed more than 48,000 people in Sub-Saharan Africa in 2008.There has however been a decrease in mortality: in 2010, there were about 9,000 deaths down from 34,000 in 1990.

The figures point to lack of consistency in the downward trend in mortality and this may be indicative of the inability to collect and analyse the causes of death in some rural communities accurately.

BIRD FLU (AVIAN FLU)

This is an infectious type of influenza that infects and spreads among birds but rarely affects humans.

There are a number of strains of the bird flu virus but 2 strains have caused more concerns lately:

- H5N1 (since 1997)
- H7N9 (since 2003)

There is no human to human transmission but there have been many people infected around the world in recent years which caused considerable concern and led to a number of deaths.

Apart from the common strains of the virus above, other strains such as H7N7,H9N2 and more recently H6N1, H10N8 and H5N6 have been identified as potentially infectious to humans though actual infection in humans have been uncommon.

Infected birds may not always be symptomatic of the disease making it difficult to isolate, treat or cull.

Bird flu can be passed between different species of affected birds such as ducks, chicken , turkeys and geese. Infection can pass between pets, wild and commercial birds.

Human transmission occurs when there is a close association and contact with birds especially those who work in the poultry industry. Individuals who keep birds as pets or hunters of wild birds are also prone to infection by bird flu.

In general, actual spread to humans follows close prolonged contact with infected bird under the following circumstances:

1. Prolonged physical or non -physical (droppings, sneezed droplets) contact with infected bird
2. Contact or inhalation of dried dust from droppings or bedding of infected birds or carcass.
3. Physical contact with live or dead infected bird
4. Inhalation or contact with sneezed droplets of infected bird
5. The butchering ,culling, slaughtering or preparation of infected bird for a meal
6. Infection by bird flu is by exposure and so visiting markets where several birds are kept in over-crowded and unsanitary conditions is a potential source of infection.

Travellers and visitors are strongly advised to avoid visiting such markets especially in endemic areas or where there has been an outbreak.

Fortunately infection by bird flu is not acquired or transmitted through cooked meat , poultry or eggs.

Prevention

Birds flu can be prevented by simple measures and paying attention to the following details:

1. If visiting countries where there has been an outbreak, do not pick up or touch birds, whether they are dead or alive.
2. Do not join in hunting or any sports involving birds in endemic regions of the world.
3. Do not visit poultry farms or live markets where birds are sold in endemic regions.
4. Do not play with, pick up or touch birds in areas where there had been an outbreak of bird flu.
5. Do not touch surfaces that have been contaminated with bird droppings.
6. Avoid eating undone or undercooked bird meat, poultry or eggs.
7. Do not bring back to your country any bird as pets, birds for commercial use, feathers or meat.
8. Remember to adopt good personal hygiene at all times such as regular washing of hands and discarding any items contaminated by birds.
9. Flocks of poultry birds should be isolated from wild birds and their waste.
10. Vehicles used in poultry industry should be regularly disinfected and not shared with other farms.
11. Use of personal protective equipment especially during outbreaks is recommended.
12. Protection should include the nose, mouth, eyes and hands as the virus can enter the body through these routes.

13. Personal protective equipment for poultry workers should include goggles, aprons, boots, boot covers, gloves and head cover.
14. Air purifying respirator should be considered during outbreak for use by poultry workers.

DENGUE FEVER

Dengue fever is caused by the dengue virus and is one of the **17 neglected tropical diseases which the World Health Organization (WHO)** has highlighted. It is an important but rarely acknowledged and recognised cause of morbidity and mortality in several tropical and subtropical countries.

The disease is transmitted through the bite of **Aedes aegypti mosquito** and other related species which are widely distributed particularly in urban areas and breed in water left in discarded containers especially cans, discarded tyres, tins and blocked drains. For this reason, A.aegypti breeds mostly in urban areas and the widespread urbanization which has taken place around the world has meant an increase in the incidence and prevalence of dengue fever in many regions. Zika virus infection follows a similar pattern which we shall come to later. The similarities in transmission should be noted.

The disease is prevalent in several tropical and subtropical countries around the world especially in:

1.South East Asia and the Far East

- India
- Pakistan
- Indonesia
- Bangladesh

- Myanmar
- Sri Lanka.
- North and South Korea
- Cambodia
- Thailand

2. Countries bordering Southern China and neighbouring Islands

- The Philippines
- Laos
- Vietnam

3. Countries in the Pacific

- Solomon Island
- New Caledonia

4. Africa

- Nigeria
- Angola
- Mozambique
- Kenya
- Ivory Coast
- Somalia
- Burkina Faso
- Senegal
- Gambia
- North Eastern Sudan adjoining the Red Sea
- Senegal
- The Gambia
- Comoros and Seychelles islands off the coast of East Africa

Dr. Usen Ikidde

5. Mexico

6. Central American countries

7. Brazil

8. North Western South American countries

- Ecuador
- Columbia
- Venezuela
- Guyana
- French Guiana

9. West Indies

10. North East Australia (Queensland) and Oceania

- Papua New Guinea.
- New Guinea

11. Middle East.

- Southern part of Yemen
- Parts of Saudi Arabia adjoining the Red Sea.

This list is not exclusive but the countries and regions mentioned above are the worst affected where dengue fever is endemic and prone to epidemics. Indeed many parts of Sub-Saharan Africa, parts of Eastern South Africa and Madagascar are affected to varying degrees, so also are the states of Florida, Alabama, Louisiana and Texas in the United States.

Symptoms of Dengue Fever.

The symptoms of dengue fever usually begin about 4-10 days after exposure-a bite by infected mosquito, and may last up to 10 days.

The symptoms may include any 2 or more of the following:

1. Fever with temperature which may be as high as 40-41 degrees C. The fever is typically biphasic: it stops only to re-start in a day or two.
2. Muscle and joint pains
3. Headache
4. A characteristic **skin rash** which resembles measles rash and best described as "islands of white in a sea of red". This picture is very typical as the skin is typically covered with reddish rash with intervening strips of normal or whitish skin (in white coloured races) In black coloured races these areas would be normal or black skin.
5. Pain behind the eyes
6. Nausea and vomiting
7. Lymphadenopathy (swollen lymph nodes)

Dengue disease may progress in a small number of patients to a life-threatening complication of **dengue haemorrhagic fever** (more likely in children and young adults) with the following additional signs and symptoms-

8. Bleeding especially from the nose, mouth and the gut
9. Very low blood pressure
10. Shock
11. Thrombocytopenia (low blood platelet count)
12. Pleural effusion (collection of fluid within the pleura in the chest)
13. Ascitis (collection of fluid within the peritoneum in the abdomen)

14. Diarrhoea
15. Itching-this may occur also in the early stage of infection.
16. Seizures
17. Fast or slow pulse may be a feature depending on the stage of infection or complications.
18. Vasculitic rash due to minute haemorrhages into the skin which fail to disappear with pressure as in meningitis rash. This causes the typical skin feature above-"islands of white in a sea of red".
19. Fatigue.
20. Complications may involve other organs such as the Central Nervous system (CNS), infection of the heart and acute liver failure-with symptomatic manifestations of dysfunctions in those organs.

The dengue virus has 5 distinct types and life long immunity is only acquired if there is re-infection with that particular type and only short term immunity to the other types. It is striking that subsequent infection by another type actually makes the situation worse by increasing the risk of complications noted above.

Fortunately for **travellers**, infectivity to the virus is low: about 80% of those infected with the virus are asymptomatic or only show mild symptoms such as low grade fever which normally stops in a few days.

The maximum length of incubation period of the virus is about 14 days, therefore, travellers who develop fever or other symptoms more than 14 days after returning home from a trip to endemic areas are unlikely to be suffering from dengue fever. Under such circumstances, other causes of fever should be sought as well.

Severe disease is more common in the following groups:

1. Babies, young children and young adults
2. Well nourished children who are overweight
3. High body mass index (BMI) -especially obese children (see 2 above)
4. Degree of viral load- People who have been highly exposed to several bites of dengue virus -carrying mosquitoes are more likely to have severe disease.
5. Africans with glucose-6-phosphate-dehydrogenase (G-6-PD) deficiency. Polymorphism or normal variations in particular genes are known to increase the likelihood of complications.

Diagnosis

Diagnosis of dengue fever is mainly based on clinical features above in individuals who are or have recently visited endemic areas.

Another useful diagnostic tool is the tourniquet test which involves the application of blood pressure cuff between the systolic and diastolic pressures for 5 minutes and counting the number of petechial haemorrhages. The likelihood of dengue disease is increased by a high number of the haemorrhages being present -more than 10-20 per square inch of skin.

It is most important to exclude other tropical and sub-tropical diseases that present with similar clinical features.

Laboratory tests may show low platelet, low white cell counts and possibly metabolic acidosis. A deranged liver function test may be evidenced by elevated aminotranferase.

When there are severe complications such as shock, this would be shown by a low blood pressure, rapid heart rate, peripheral vascular collapse and delayed capillary refill and cold extremities especially in children.

In more advanced centres, when dengue haemorrhagic shock has ensued, ultrasound scan is likely to demonstrate pleural effusion and ascitis (see above under symptoms and clinical features).

The definitive diagnosis of dengue fever can be confirmed in the laboratory by identification of dengue virus in cell cultures, nucleic acid detection, viral antigen or specific antibodies detection methods.

Prevention

Prevention of dengue fever is important as there are no effective vaccines to fight off the disease.

Prevention of breeding, proliferation and protection from bites of the vector-Aedes Aegypti mosquito form the bedrock on which prevention depends.

To this end the following methods (in addition to WHO recommendations of integrated Vector Control programme) should be adopted:

1. Get rid of sources of open stagnant water especially by removal of tins, pots, cans, other containers, discarded tyres and closure of open drains. In this way the habitat of the mosquito vector, Aedes aegypti, is eliminated.
2. By use of insecticides
3. Enviromental modification by reducing the sources of open collection of standing water is preferred to the use of insecticides as the latter may not be effective after prolonged use due to resistance to the

insecticides. In addition to the problem of resistance, there are environmental implications to humans, animals and plants. These are other considerations for a change in strategy.

4. Use of long sleeve shirts, socks, boots and long trousers are other ways of preventing exposure to mosquito bites.
5. Use of well-fitted mosquito net
6. Use of insect repellent: DEET is considered to be quite effective.
7. The first dengue fever vaccine has been produced in Mexico and received approval in December 2015 and expected to be in use by 2016. The vaccine which was developed by the French company Sanofi has only about 60% effectiveness and is limited to people aged 9-45 years. This limitation in scope, age and efficacy shows that there is still a lot of work to be done in order to ensure universal use. However, this is one example where "half bread is better than none".
8. Research attempts are on going to infect the A.aegypti mosquito population with bacteria of the genus Wolbachia to make the mosquitoes at least partially resistant to the dengue virus. So far, the artificially induced infection has been successful but there is uncertainty whether the naturally acquired infection would do the same.
9. Vector control is important and is the bedrock in the prevention of this disease. To this end, in order to reduce the mosquito population, guppy fish or copepods have been introduced into standing pool of water to eat the mosquito lavae and thus stop their development into adult mosquitoes.
10. Another novel research has been the "creation" of a genetically modified male A. aegypti mosquitoes which when released mate with the females but

render the offspring incapable of flying and thus cannot get to human population and bite.
11. Attempts at development of antiviral medication specifically for dengue fever has so far proved abortive.

In addition to the above measures, **The World Health Organization (WHO)** recommends an Integrated Vector Control programme which consists of 5 elements:

1. Advocacy, social mobilization and legislation to ensure that public health bodies and communities are strengthened.
2. It recommends collaboration between the health and other sectors (public and private).
3. It advocates an integrated approach to disease control to maximize use of resources.
4. It also recommends evidence- based decision making to ensure any interventions are targeted appropriately.
5. WHO advises adequate capacity building to ensure an adequate response to the local situation.

The importance of the prevention of dengue fever is the observation every year on June 15 of international Anti-Dengue Day. Three Asian countries have so far taken the lead in this respect:

1. Jakarta, Indonesia in 2011,
2. Yangon, Myanmar in 2012 and
3. Vietnam in 2013.

The aim of Anti-dengue Day is to increase awareness of the disease and the mobilization of available resources for control and the prevention of this "neglected disease".

Treatment of Dengue Fever

There are no anti viral vaccines or specific medication for dengue except the recently developed vaccine in Mexico which has not yet been widely used. See above. The management of this disease is therefore symptomatic and the following measures are considered useful:

1. Painkillers and antipyretic medications to manage pain and fever-Acetaminophen (Paracetamol) is usually enough. NSAID like Ibuprofen should be avoided as it could cause more bleeding.
2. Maintenace of fluid balance by oral rehydration therapy or intravenous fluids
3. Complicated or severe cases require intensive care management with emphasis on fluid replacement titrated to urinary output.
4. Regular monitoring of vital signs especially blood pressure, pulse and temperature should be carried out.
5. Blood transfusion may be necessary as indicated in the face decreasing **haematocrit** rather than waiting for haemoglobin results. Packed red or whole blood are usually recommended.

The Global Problem and Epidemiology of Dengue Fever Disease

1. The disease infects 50-528 million people yearly.
2. Dengue fever affects people in more than 110 countries world wide.
3. Dengue fever was first identified and confirmed in South East Asia.
4. About 12 countries in South East Asia are affected.
5. In 2000s, there were an estimated 3 million infections and 6,000 deaths in South East Asia.

6. Dengue fever in South East Asia has now spread to Southern China, Oceania, Southern United States and poised to threaten Europe.
7. Currently there are about 500,000 hospital admissions a year and approximately 25,000 deaths due to dengue fever or its complications.
8. More than 22 countries are affected by Dengue fever in Africa involving nearly a quarter of the population.
9. The world-wide distribution makes dengue one of the commonest vector-borne diseases.
10. Dengue is still regarded as being mostly an urban disease and the rapid urbanisation in developing countries has made worse an already bad situation.
11. There has been a 30 fold increase in dengue fever between 1960 and 2010.This has been attributable to increased international travel, rapid urbanization, population growth, global warming and failure of governments, health institutions and international organizations to appreciate the severity and magnitude of the problem and failure to tackle it head-on.
12. The tropics and subtropical regions bear the brunt of this problem.
13. About 2.5 billion people live in the areas affected by dengue fever; 70% of these are in Asia and Oceania.
14. Dengue disease is the second most common cause of fever in travellers returning from developing countries: The first position is still occupied by malaria.
15. Despite its pre-eminent position as a cause of fever, morbidity and mortality, dengue disease is hardly known or mentioned in many affected communities, medical literature, healthcare settings, some governments and international healthcare organizations.

16. It is for this reason that the **World Health Organization (WHO)** has rightly placed it in the number one position as **one of the 17 neglected tropical diseases.** See chapter six.
17. Dengue fever is also the most common viral disease transmitted by arthropods. Note that malaria is not a viral disease :that is why dengue occupies the number one position.
18. Though the disease is transmitted to humans in urban areas by Aedes aegypti mosquito,but in rural settings and forests of South East Asia and Africa, the transmission is also effected by female Aedes mosquitoes belonging to other species, not necessarily A.aegypti. Lower primates in these forests, rather than humans, form the main reservoir or intermediary host to continue the cycle.

HAND, FOOT AND MOUTH DISEASE

This is a viral infection that mostly affects young children but may also affect older children and adults. It is caused by an enterovirus especially-

coxsackie virus A16,A6,A10 and enterovirus 71.

It is known that the latter carries a higher risk of serious complications.

It is important to state here that human form of this disease-hand, foot and mouth disease has no relationship with foot and mouth disease that affects animals especially cattle, sheep and pigs. **Humans cannot therefore catch the animal form of the disease.**

Dr. Usen Ikidde

The typical incubation period (the time between exposure to the disease and start of symptoms) is 3- 6 days.

In the UK and many other countries it doesn't seem to pose a serious threat to children's health but that has not been the case in some Far East countries.

The clinical features of the this infection are typified by the following:

1. There is a high temperature of about 38-39 C
2. Loss of appetite
3. A cough
4. Sore throat
5. Abdominal pain
6. Nausea
7. Vomiting
8. Tiredness or out of sorts.

The early symptoms tend to disappear within 48 hours.

After about 24-48 hours ulcers are heralded in as follows:

9. **Mouth ulcers**-these are small red spots inside the mouth, usually on the tongue, inside of the cheeks and on the gums. The spots become small sores and then rapidly develop into large mouth ulcers which are greyish- yellow in colour and surrounded by red round area of tissue. There may be as many as 10 of these ulcers.

The ulcer may be quite painful especially in children where it makes drinking, sucking, eating and swallowing quite uncomfortable. The child may then refuse to drink or eat altogether and discomfort in swallowing saliva may lead to dribbling.

Under normal circumstances, the mouth ulcers heal and disappear within a period of about one week

10. The appearance of **mouth ulcers** are accompanied closely by **hand and foot disease**.

The commonest areas for the appearance of hand and foot diseases are the fingers, palms of the hand and soles of the feet. There may also be involvement of the groin and buttocks. The spots are usually ovoid or elliptical in shape, about 0.5 cm with a dark- grey centre.

The spots may blister and so become painful and tender to touch. Pricking or bursting the blisters easily spreads the virus infection to others, so breaking open the blisters should be resisted. Like mouth ulcers the hand and foot spots and blisters tend to last for only about 10 days before they disappear.

Most children with hand, foot and mouth disease do not need any special medical attention, but this may be necessary when the child shows certain features:

1. The child's condition deteriorates due to high fever or persistent spots.
2. The child refuses or is unable to eat and drink.
3. The child's nappies are unusually dry which shows he/she is not passing enough urine.
4. The child shows other signs of dehydration such as a dry mucous membrane or wrinkling of the skin due to poor skin tone.
5. The child shows no symptomatic improvement or is getting worse after a week.
6. The child displays behavioural or personality changes.
7. Fits or seizures

Dr. Usen Ikidde

Spread of hand, foot and mouth disease.

This viral infection is spread by direct contact in the following ways:

1. By direct contact with burst blisters
2. Direct contact with mucus
3. Contact with infected saliva
4. Contact with faeces of infected person.

Complications

A few people may have complications such as:

1. Meningitis (inflammation of the covering of the spinal cord or brain)
2. Encephalitis (inflammation of the brain)
3. Paralysis
4. Pleural effusion (fluid in the lung space)
5. Carditis (inflammation of the heart)
6. There may be bleeding into the lungs.
7. Very occasionally toenail and fingernail losses have been reported.

Prevention

There is no vaccine available for this viral disease but efforts are being made to develop a vaccine in the future.

Hand, foot and mouth disease is a very contagious infection and prevention revolves around stopping the modes of spread through nasopharyngeal discharges or secretions, direct contact, nasal mucus and saliva.

The following measures should be observed:

1. Avoid direct contact with infected children or adults.
2. Proper cleaning and disinfection of contaminated surfaces
3. Keeping infected children off school
4. Regular hand hygiene
5. Personal hygiene during the infective period

Treatment

Treatment of hand, foot and mouth disease is symptomatic: fever, pain and discomfort should be managed with painkillers such as Acetaminophen

(Paracetamol).

There are no specific medications or vaccines for the treatment or prevention of hand, foot and mouth disease. In most cases the disease runs a short course of 7-10 days after which the symptoms disappear.

A few people who develop complications need to be admitted into hospital especially those with meningitis, encephalitis, carditis or pleural effusion.

A brief History and Epidemiology of Hand, foot and Mouth Disease

There have been major outbreaks, morbidity and mortality due to hand, foot and mouth disease in several countries in the Far East. Some of the recorded ones are as follows:

1. Taiwan in 1998 with an estimated 1.5 million cases affecting mostly children with 78 deaths and 405 severe complications

2. China in March 2008 with 42 deaths and about 25 000 people affected
3. Singapore in April the same year 2600 cases
4. Vietnam in the same year with 2300 cases and eleven deaths
5. Mongolia in the same year with 1600 cases
6. Brunei in the same year with 1053 cases
7. China again in March/April 2009 in the Eastern Shandon Province with 17 deaths and the neighbouring Henan Province with 18 children's deaths.
8. There were 115000 reported cases in China that year with a total mortality of 50 and 773 severe cases which occurred from January to April.
9. China 2010 there was another outbreak with 40 deaths and 70,756 recorded cases all in the southern provinces.
10. China 2011.Between January and October, WHO reported the drop to 1,340,259 by about 300,000 from 2010 (1,654,866).
11. United States of America in 2011 where the California Department of Public Health identified the virus caused by the A6 coxsackie virus, a stronger variant which caused an unusual complication in children with nail loss.
12. Alabama,USA in 2012 there was an outbreak of an usual type and unusual season of occurrence of the disease which affected mostly older children and teenagers. Some of these people were admitted to hospital but fortunately there were no deaths recorded.
13. Cambodia 2012.Despite doubts, laboratory tests showed that 52 of the 59 children who died, the test of most of the children were positive of hand, foot and mouth disease virus. WHO report attested to this fact.

14. China up till 2012.There were 1520274 cases of hand, foot and mouth disease with 431 deaths.
15. Syria early 2015.More than 200 cases of the disease were reported.
16. New Zealand 1957.This is where the first cases of hand, foot and mouth disease were first reported and described.

LEPTOSPIROSIS

Leptospirosis is an infection caused by the bacteria-Leptospira.The disease is spread by animals, mostly rodents, and transmitted to humans by their urine which has contaminated the soil or water when this comes into contact with man through the mouth, eyes, nose or a break on the skin.

In most cases the infection is unnoticed or the symptoms may be quite subtle or wrongly attributable to other infections or diseases.

The following animals are known to carry leptospira bacteria:

1. Rodents-particularly rats
2. Pigs
3. Cattle
4. Dogs
5. Horses
6. Sheep
7. Deer
8. Rabbit
9. Hedgehogs
10. Cows
11. Racoons
12. Skunk

13. Opposums
14. Rarely domestic pets like pet rat
15. Banded Mongoose-in Africa.

Infection is generally uncommon but certain people belonging to the following groups and occupations or who regularly engage in some leisure activities are more prone to leptospirosis infection. These are:

1. You regularly deal with animals in any capacity which involves touching live or dead animals especially if that is your occupation which therefore exposes you to regular and close contact with animals.
2. You are a farmer
3. A Vet
4. You take part in water sports (This why this infection is relevant to tourist or travellers)
5. Fishermen
6. If you come into contact with contaminated water, soil or sewage
7. You have suffered a rodent bite
8. Drinking contaminated water
9. Physical contact with blood or tissue of infected animals.

Certain outdoor activities which bring you in contact with contaminated soil, water or sewage such as:

10. Camping in rural areas (This is relevant to travellers and tourist)
11. Sailing (Relevant to holiday makers or tourist)
12. Swimming (Important for Tourist)
13. Canoeing (Tourist and holiday makers)
14. Caving. (Holiday makers and tourist)
15. Rafting (Also important for tourist and holiday makers to note)

16. Potholing (Same as above for tourist)
17. Infection is more likely following a flood where there is widespread contamination with infected soil, water and sewage material.

Leptospirosis occurs more commonly in tropical and subtropical regions of the world especially in:

1. South East Asia.
2. India
3. China
4. Australia
5. Africa
6. South and Central America
7. The West Indies.

Notably, human to human transmission of leptospirosis is very rare.

Signs and symptoms.

There may be no signs or symptoms of leptospirosis infection or may be so subtle that they are virtually unnoticeable or may be mild, but in about 10% of cases there may be quite severe and involve some organs of the body especially the liver, brain ,eyes, the gastrointestinal tract, kidney, musculoskeletal and respiratory systems.

In severe cases when there is involvement of the liver leading to jaundice, kidney failure and bleeding, the infection is called **Weil's disease.**

Here are some of the signs and symptoms:

1. Headache
2. Muscles pain especially in the calves and lower back

3. Fever
4. Nausea
5. Vomiting
6. Loss of appetite
7. Cough
8. Conjunctivitis
9. Bleeding from the lung may manifest as haemoptysis (coughing out blood)
10. Jaundice due to liver infection
11. Kidney failure
12. Swelling of the hands, ankles and feet
13. shortness of breath
14. Chest pains
15. Meningitis
16. Encephalitis
17. Fits

The mild symptoms usually develop within a week to 2 weeks after exposure and last for 5-7 days. The severe signs and symptoms due to complications may continue unless there is a medical intervention and could result in death.

Prevention

This infection can largely be prevented by taking all the necessary precautions if you belong to the high risk groups above especially those whose occupation involves close contact with animals.

Sewage workers should particularly take precautions by wearing boots, gloves and adequately covering all cuts on their skin. It is also important to prevent contact with sewage material especially to the eyes, mouth and nose.

People on vacations/ holidays abroad in infected regions, should where possible avoid coming into contact with or exposure to rivers, ponds and lakes. Those who engage in sports or leisure activities where contact is inevitable should take adequate precautions necessary to minimize or preferable prevent any contact or exposure to any possible source of infection.

Treatment

The initial treatment is symptomatic. Pain and fever are relieved by simple analgesia such as Acetaminophen (Paracetamol).

The definitive treatment is with antibiotics such as Doxycycline or Penicillin. It is important to finish the course of your antibiotics to prevent recurrence.

Severe Leptospirosis infection and Weil's disease usually require admission to hospital and treatment with intravenous antibiotics.

In severe cases where there are organ involvement and failure, treatment is directed accordingly to the particular problem. For instance, dialysis is required in renal failure. A ventilator will assist in severe breathing problems.

In severe cases where there is nausea and vomiting or renal failure, correction of fluid and electrolyte imbalance are required. Intravenous fluids should be given as necessary.

Admission is mandatory during pregnancy as the fetus may also be affected and the monitoring of both mother and baby should be carried out to reduce the risk to both.

Dr. Usen Ikidde

MENINGOCOCCAL DISEASE (Meningococcus)

This is caused by the bacterium **Neisseria meningitides**. This infection is a cause of **meningitis** and blood infection-**sepsis,** both of which carry high morbidity and mortality.

Meningococcal Disease can be prevented by vaccination. Neisseria meningitides is harmless to many people but to others, it is a serious source of infection to the blood stream and colonizes the entire body but particularly the brain and limbs causing serious illness.

Transmission can be effected through saliva e.g. by kissing and also by close prolonged contact with an infected individual.

The symptoms depend on the effect of the disease (meningitis or sepsis).Meningitis is the infection of the membranes of the brain and spinal cord (the meninges).When it causes **meningitis** the following symptoms may occur:

1. High fever with cold hands and feet
2. Drowsiness
3. Vomiting
4. Irritability
5. Confusion
6. Difficulty in waking up from sleep
7. Distinctive rash
8. Pale and blotchy skin
9. Severe headache
10. Photophobia (sensitivity to light)
11. Neck stiffness
12. Convulsions or seizures

Babies and young children under 5 are more prone to meningitis than adults and the symptoms above depend on the age of the child. Adults are not exempt from this infection.

Meningitis is a medical emergency and should be treated as such when some of the symptoms above become evident.

In meningococcal septicaemia, the glass test should be performed by pressing the side of a clear glass against the skin and in positive cases the rash would not disappear as in other types of skin rash.(See also Dengue fever with similar outcome).

Viral meningitis is usually less serious than meningococcal meningitis with symptoms of fever,headche and generally feeling unwell. In severe cases there may also be neck stiffness , nausea, vomiting, muscle and joint pains, photophobia and diarrhoea. Viral meningitis does not usually cause blood poisoning (sepsis)

Sepsis (blood poisoning) Meningococcal disease can also cause sepsis. Like meningitis, this is also a medical emergency.

In "blood poisoning", the body's immune system is overwhelmed by an infection which spreads rapidly in the blood stream and sets off a number of reactions leading to organ failure.Organ failure is due to profound decrease in blood pressure (hypotension) leading to a reduction in blood supply to vital organs - the heart, brain, kidney etc . This can lead to multiple organ failure and death unless treatment is instituted as soon as possible.

It is therefore most important to seek medical help as soon as the symptoms of sepsis are apparent.

Dr. Usen Ikidde

The signs and symptoms include:

1. High fever
2. Fast breathing
3. Shivering.
4. Hypotension
5. Tachycardia (fast pulse rate)
6. Dizziness
7. Disorientation
8. Confusion
9. Nausea and vomiting
10. Cold pale, clammy and mottled skin.
11. Diarrhoea
12. Slurred speech
13. Severe muscle pains
14. Decrease in urine output
15. Loss of consciousness

There is some overlap in the symptoms of meningitis and sepsis since the latter may progress to the former and vice versa. Besides, both can co-exist.

Sepsis may also be caused by other bacteria especially the gram negative bacteria. Sepsis is more likely if you have recently had a bowel or urinary tract operation, had an injury or infection. Sepsis may also arise de novo or from other unsuspected sources of infection.

The most important message is to attend the Emergency Department of your nearest hospital immediately sepsis is suspected by calling the ambulance especially if the patient is already unconscious as private transport may be unsuitable under such circumstances.

Meningococcal disease may also lead to other types of infections including meningococcal pneumonia, pericarditis(infection of the covering of the heart) as part of septic pericarditis, myocarditis,pharyngitis,conjunctivitis, septic arthritis following disseminated meningococcal infection, osteomyelitis (bone infection) and urethral infection.

Prevention

Different strains or serotypes of Neisseria meningitides are recognized as A, B, C,Y, and W135.These subtypes are responsible for nearly all cases of meningococcal disease.

The prevalence of each of these groups differs from country to country and quite often depends on the age they are more likely to affect.

In the UK almost all childhood meningococcal disease are caused by the the subgroups B and C. Childhood immunization is therefore directed at these 2 subgroups.

The disease declines with age. Except exposed individuals, immunodeficiency, travel to endemic regions and individual country requirements,immunization is generally not recommended for those over 25 years of age in the UK.

Routine immunization is given to children at 2 months(group B), 3 months (group C),booster at 4 months (group B). Another booster at 12-13 months is sometimes given.At 14 years, vaccination is given against subgroups C and W (men C and W).

Vaccination (Men W vaccine) should be given at 13-18 years to those individuals who are at risk of infection .Those at risk include the following :

1. Travellers to endemic regions

2. Teenagers and adults who share dormitories as in boarding schools
3. Health care workers and people who are exposed to infected individuals
4. Asplenia are- People whose spleens have been surgically removed, congenitally absent or have non-functioning spleen.
5. Those with complement or immunodeficiency.

Visitors to endemic countries are advised to have their immunization before embarking on their journey. They are also advised to check that country's immunization requirements several weeks before travelling.

Travellers to Saudi Arabia, in particular are required to have proof of tetravalent vaccination against meningococcal subgroups A,C,W135 and Y.

Travellers to Sub-Saharan Africa, Asia and the Indian Subcontinent where the disease is mostly endemic are advised to have immunization even if there is no specific requirement by the country concerned.

Treatment

Meningococcal disease is a medical emergency and admission to hospital should not be delayed.

The definitive treatment is to give Benzyl penicillin 1200 mg intravenously or intramuscularly for adults if there there is no history of penicillin allergy. Half this dose should be given to children aged 1-9 years of age and half this (a quarter of adult dose) to children aged below 1 year of age. Intramuscular injection is preferred for children.

Cefotaxime is the alternative antibiotic for those with penicillin allergy.

Investigations in hospital should include blood culture and sensitivity, a full blood count (FBC), urea and electrolytes (U & Es).

A lumber puncture and cerebrospinal (CSF) fluid sent for microscopy, culture and sensitivity, glucose and any evidence of raised intracranial pressure should be noted.

Supportive therapy in hospital should include intravenous fluids and may include treatment of complications such as renal failure by dialysis and anticoagulants for disseminated intravascular coaguation.

Corticosteroids may be given to reduce complications such as hearing loss and neurological complications.

Children should be reassessed by the Paediatrician and any complications noted and adequately managed.

Ciprofloxacin or rimfampicin should be given to close contacts such as siblings, those in the same dormitory as well as close friends who had come into close physical contact with the individual.

MURRAY VALLEY ENCEPHALITIS VIRUS

This is a mosquito-borne viral infection spread by the mosquito, culex annulirostris in Northern Australia and Papua New Guinea.

Birds act as reservoirs or amplifiers for this infection. The principal viral cycle therefore exists between birds and the mosquito vectors which transmit the infection to humans. There is no human to human transmission of this virus.

The water birds are migratory with the tendency to move to different parts of Australia including the south east where the Murray-Darling river outbreak occurred in 1951 in the Murray valley. The virus was isolated from human samples during the outbreak in this region and the name was changed from Australian encephalitis to Murray valley encephalitis.

It is estimated that only about 1:1000 people who are bitten by the mosquito become infected by this vector-borne virus. Besides, not all the mosquitoes carry the virus. Infection is more likely during periods of heavy rainfall and flooding. This provides ideal conditions for the breeding of mosquitoes.

Many people who get bitten by mosquitoes and get the virus don't show any symptoms which may include:

1. A high fever
2. Severe headache
3. Stiffness of the neck
4. Fits or seizures
5. Drowsiness
6. Coma

Prevention is by:

- preventing any conditions which aid the breeding of mosquitoes
- protecting yourself from mosquitoe bites
- avoiding being outside when mosquitoes are very active especially before dawn and sunset.

- wearing adequate clothing that helps to protect against possible mosquito bites.To this end, light coloured clothing , long sleeve shirts, long trousers and socks should be worn.
- mosquito repellent containing DEET (diethyl toluamide) on exposed areas of the skin has been found to be useful. In children, this should be rubbed or sprayed on clothing rather than the skin.
- use of mosquito nets which should be carefully tucked in below the mattress and should have no holes.

Diagnosis

Diagnosis is made by:

- clinical symptoms
- clinical signs
- blood test

Treatment

There is no specific treatment for MVE. Treatment is supportive or symptomatic and should include: treatment or management of fever, headache, seizures and coma.

It is worth remembering that most people who are infected recover fully whilst a few others require immediate and long term treatment and support due to brain damage.

Dr. Usen Ikidde

PNEUMOCOCCAL DISEASE (Streptococcus pneumonia)

This is caused by Streptococcus pneumoniae bacteria which cause several infections that range from mild to severe.

Despite the name in bracket, Streptococcus pneumoniae is responsible for several other disease entities other than pneumonia.

According to the World Health Organization (WHO), **pneumococcal disease is the most preventable cause of death by vaccination in infants and children under 5 years of age.**

As noted above, Streptococcal pneumonia may be responsible for the following diseases or infections:

1. Pneumonia (lung infection)
2. Sepsis (severe blood infection often referred to as "blood poisoning")
3. Meningitis (inflammation of the lining of the spinal cord/ brain)
4. Otitis media (middle ear infection)
5. Conjunctivitis (eye infection)
6. Sinusitis (infection of the sinuses -hollow cavities filled with air in bone found around the face, nose and head)
7. Bronchitis (inflammation/ infection of air passages to the lung)
8. Bacteraemia (mild entry of the bacteria into the blood stream, controlled by immune response. Compare sepsis in number 2 above.
9. Osteomylitis (bone infection)
10. Septic arthritis (joint infection by bacteria)

11. Peritonitis (inflammation/infection of the lining of the abdomen)
12. Pericarditis (inflammation/infection of the outer lining of the heart)
13. Endocarditis.(inflammation/infection of the inner lining of the heart)
14. Cellulitis (inflammation of the skin)
15. Brain abcess (infection of the brain)

Symptoms of pneumococcal disease depend largely on severity, age, immunity and which of the organs above are affected. Let me give some examples as follows:

1. **Pneumococcal pneumonia.** The symptoms here depend on the age of the patient and the following may be apparent especially in children:

- fever
- cough
- rapid or difficulty in breathing
- chest pain in both adults and older children
- confusion and reduced alertless especially in the elderly.

Symptoms of pneumococcal meningitis

May include:

- Fever
- Neck stiffness
- Photophobia (discomfort on looking at bright light)
- Headache
- Seizures or fits
- Vomiting especially in children
- Refusal to eat or drink mostly also in children.

Dr. Usen Ikidde

Symptoms and signs of pneumococcal sepsis may include the following:

- High fever
- Low temperature may occur instead and lead to chills and shivering
- Refusal to feed (in children)
- Cold clammy skin due to decreased blood supply to the skin as well as the chills and shivering noted above
- Drowsiness
- Feeling very unwell
- Rapid pulse or heart rate due to increased demand on the heart to pump blood faster to oxygenate all parts of the body especially the vital organs; the lungs, heart itself, the brain and kidneys.
- Decreased urine output which may be due to the effect on the kidney and other vital organs above due to overwhelming infection and may lead to multiple organ failure. May also result from excessive diarrhoea and vomiting leading to dehydration, low blood pressure and limited amount of fluid to the kidneys.
- Nausea, vomiting and diarrhoea may occur as explained above; these may be due to multiple organ effect of sepsis which also affects the gastrointestinal tract .
- Dizziness especially in the adult patient which may be due to low blood pressure and consequently less blood supply to vital organs such as the brain and inner ear. Severe dizziness or vertigo may precede septic shock.
- Changes in mental state as explained above may be due to effect on the brain by overwhelming infection and decreased blood pressure and oxygenated blood.
- slurred speech for reasons above

- severe muscle pain
- breathlessness due to increased demand for oxygenated blood in which the body reacts via the brain to increase breathing to try and compensate for the decreasing oxygen saturation.
- There is decreasing or loss of consciousness due to decreased blood supply to the brain and inability to perform its functions including the maintenance of consciousness.

Symptoms and signs of otitis media may include:

- ear pain
- fever
- excessive crying by the child
- redness and swelling of the ear drum

In osteomylitis, there may be:

- excessive crying due to discomfort
- bone pains
- refusal to use the affected limb such as reluctance to walk, crawl or stand.

Spread

Entry is through the nose and mouth in the same way as flu or cold. Direct contact is by tiny droplets during coughing or sneezing. The tiny droplets contain streptococcus pneumoniae bacteria which are then breathed by others who become infected.

Indirect spread occurs when an infected person transfers infected material to shared objects e.g. door handle, keys, computer which others touch inadvertently and transfer to their mouths or noses and then become infected.

Diagnosis is based on:

- history of contact
- clinical history
- clinical examination
- positive blood culture

Prevention

Prevention is by:

- proper washing of hands by infected people before touching shared articles which others are likely to handle
- Hand hygiene should be by soap and water and if possible by sanitizer which contains at least 60% alcohol.
- Avoid touching your mouth and nose.
- Always cover your mouth and nose during sneezing or coughing with proper tissue paper not with your hands. This should prevent the spread by droplets and transfer to others. The tissue paper should be carefully disposed off so as not to act as another source of infection to others.
- The bed rock to prevention lies in the active vaccination with pneumococcal vaccines which are given as follows:

1. In the UK, babies are vaccinated at 2,4 and between 12-13 months of age with pneumococcal conjugate vaccine (PCV) which contains 13 strains of the inactivated bacteria.
2. Adults aged 65 and over are given a single dose of the pneumococcal polysaccharide vaccine (PPV) which contains 23 strains of the inactivated bacteria.

3. People with conditions (see above) which make them susceptible to pneumococcal infection or with lowered immunity status are given either a single one off dose or 5 yearly depending on the severity of the underlying medical condition.

The PCV and PPC vaccines are both inactive bacteria with no live organisms and so should not cause the disease which they are given to protect against.

Travellers who have not been vaccinated should avail themselves of vaccination before travelling abroad on vacation/ holidays where they may come into contact with infected people or contaminated shared objects or utensils.

Treatment depends on the severity,age,parts of the body affected or type of infection but generally should include the following measures:

- rest
- taking plenty of fluids
- painkillers such as paracetamol
- antibiotics for invasive infection preferably with admission to hospital especially children and the elderly.
- swabs should be taken for definitive diagnosis and for culture and sensitivity of the bacteria.

RABIES

This is a serious viral infection transmitted to human through the bite of infected animals.Rabies virus targets the brain and the entire central nervous system.

Rabies can be prevented by vaccination and by prompt treatment after exposure before the development of symptoms, otherwise rabies infection is almost invariably fatal.

More than 95% of mortality due to rabies are in Africa and Asia and usually due to a bite by an infected dog. The other 5% are found in other continents and due to transmission by bats, occasional dog bite or by other animals. **Unvaccinated travellers** may also be bitten by dogs in these areas before travelling back home, sometimes unaware of the serious consequences of their exposure.

Despite the higher number of rabies cases in Africa and Asia, rabies is present but not endemic in 150 countries world wide and sporadic cases do occur in these countries.

Rabies virus can be transmitted by a bite, scratch,or a lick by several animals especially:

- dogs
- bats
- raccoons
- foxes
- jackals
- cats
- mongooses
- monkeys
- skunks
- cattle
- wolves
- coyotes
- bears
- groundhogs
- weasels

The bite, scratch or lick by an infected animal may infect human by entering broken skin, eye, mouth or nose. Spitting by an infected animal to the skin or face may also lead to infection.

Rabies virus has the propensity to multiply and spread to nerve endings and from there, travel to the spinal cord and ultimately to the brain (CNS). Once in the brain, it spreads rapidly to vital organs including the kidneys, lungs and salivary glands. Death may follow 2-10 days after the commencement of symptoms.

The usual incubation period (time between the animal bite to the development of symptoms) is 1-3 months but may be as early as 4 days or as long as one year.

Symptoms of rabies may include any of the following:

- fever
- photophobia (sensitivity to light)
- hydrophobia (fear of water)
- confusion
- aggressive behaviour
- anxiety
- violent movements of the body
- inability to move some parts of the body
- insomnia (inability to sleep)
- partial paralysis
- terror
- hallucinations
- loss of consciousness

Diagnosis can only be made after the development of symptoms (see above for symptoms) By that time, diagnosis is only made for theoretical reasons as the potential for cure is virtually non-existent.

Other tests may include skin biopsy of affected area, blood and salivary tests.

Prevention: Pre-exposure vaccination is the key to prevention. This is usually recommended to the following groups of people:

- travellers to endemic areas of the world with limited medical care
- those who work with potentially infected animals
- veterinary surgeons
- those who regularly make contact with potentially infected animals
- people who work with or handle bats (bat handlers).

Treatment:

As noted above "prevention is better than cure". This well known axiom applies even more to rabies. Do not wait for a cure: go for prevention by pre-exposure vaccination. There is no cure after the development of symptoms of rabies, however cure can still be effected after exposure before symptoms develop by adopting the following measures:

1. Wash the area /wound/ leak by the suspected animal thoroughly with soap and running water.
2. The use of providone iodine may help to reduce the number of viruses in the wound.
3. The wound should be left open with a simple dressing only. Stitching may expose the nerve endings to the virus.
4. Seek expert medical advice.
5. Post exposure course of rabies vaccine is sine qua non. For unimmunised person or those who have had incomplete immunisation, 5 doses of rabies

vaccine should be given over one month on days 0,3,7,14 and 28-30 days.
6. Rabies immunoglobulin is also required. This is usually useful as it provides an already made antirabies antibodies which neutralise the rabies virus and thus prevent the spread to nerves and other organs. A single dose is required either immediately or within 7 days after the start of active immunization with rabies vaccine.

RIFT VALLEY FEVER

This is a viral disease that affects cattle and sheep and transmitted to humans through the following ways:

- the handling of infected animals
- from infected blood of animals
- drinking infected milk
- eating undercooked meat
- airborne
- bites from infected mosquitoes

Rift Valley Fever (RVF) was first discovered in the Rift valley in Kenya in the early 1900s. The virus is spread to livestock through the bites of infected mosquitoes and is also another method of spread to humans (see above) and usually follows a period of heavy rainfall providing breeding ground for mosquitoes.

RVF causes high mortality in young animals and abortions in pregnant female livestock and this unexplained abortions is often the first clue as to the diagnosis.

Rift Valley Fever is zoonotic (able to spread to humans via contact with infected animals).

Dr. Usen Ikidde

Symptoms and signs in animals include:

- vomiting
- diarrhoea
- lethargy
- weakness
- anorexia
- lymphadenopathy
- abortions
- death in young animals

Symptoms and signs in humans include:

- fever
- flu like symptoms
- back pain
- weight loss
- dizziness
- severe headaches
- And in severe cases :
- eye disease
- meningitis (inflammation of the covering of the spinal cord or brain)
- encephalitis (inflammation of the brain)
- haemorrhage (bleeding)
- permanent loss of vision (blindness)
- confusion
- liver disease
- bleeding from the gums
- kidney disease
- There are a number of animals that are the amplifying hosts to the virus and include the following:
- sheep
- goat
- cattle

- Afrcan buffalo
- water buffalo
- camels
- wild African rodents
- rats (Rattus rattus)
- some gray squirrels
- hamsters

The virus is spread by Aedes and Culex mosquitoes; anopheles mosquito has also be implicated.

Rift Valley Fever is endemic in Kenya and surrounding East African countries but sporadic cases or major outbreaks have also beeen reported in the following countries:

- Egypt
- Yemen
- Saudi Arabia
- Some sub-Saharan African countries
- Madagascar
- Somalia
- Sudan
- South Africa

Mortality rate in humans may be as high as 50% in severe cases but overall mortality is only about 1-2 %.

Prevention.

The most important measures include the following :

1. Control mosquito population by prevention of breeding- eliminating breeding sites.
2. Mosquito spray with insecticide

3. Prevent mosquito bites by avoiding breeding grounds and areas of high mosquito population.
4. Wearing long sleeve shirts and trousers
5. Use of mosquito nets which are properly tucked in below the mattress
6. Personal protection from contact with infected animals by use of surgical masks and gloves if handling animals in endemic areas
7. Travellers should preferably avoid visiting endemic areas during periods of high infectivity which would usually follow prolonged period of heavy rainfall.
8. Animal and human vaccine are available and should be used. Travellers should avail themselves of this vaccine before travelling to endemic areas especially those who make contact with potentially infected animals and animal products.
9. There should be disease surveillance in cattle and management protocol before, during and after outbreak in endemic and holoendemic areas.

Diagnosis is based on:

1. Symptoms and signs of the disease especially in endemic areas following a period of heavy rainfall, contact with infected animals and mosquito bites
2. Antibodies in the blood of animals or humans
3. Isolation of Rift Valley virus in the blood of infected animal or humans.

Treatment

There is no specific treatment for RVF. Treatment is symptomatic and consists of the management of specific problems as they arise, such as fever, back pain, eye disease, haemorrhage, kidney disease, meningoencephalitis etc.

RUBELLA (German Measles)

This is a viral infection that used to be common in children which has now been considerably reduced in incidence with the routine introduction of MMR vaccine (Measles, Mumps and Rubella).Left untreated, the condition is mild and usually improves within one to two weeks.

Spread: Rubella spreads through droplets in the same way as cold or flu. When an infected person coughs, sneezes or talks, the droplets are released into the air. One becomes infected by coming into contact with the droplets and could take up to 2-3 weeks for the symptoms to develop although infectivity to other people actually starts up to a week before the development of symptoms and up to 3-4 days after the appearance of the rash.

During this stage it is advisable for children to stay away from school, playground and avoid making contact with other children and pregnant women.

Symptoms:

- skin rash consisting of small spots which is red - pink in colour
- fever
- enlargement of lymph glands
- painful aching joints especially in adults
- flu like symptoms especially cold, cough,,runny nose,watery eyes and sore throat
- loss of appetite
- tiredness or lethargy

The incubation period (the time between exposure and development of symptoms) is usually 2-3 weeks. Some exposed people show no symptoms at all. Others have rashes or spots which start behind the ears and spread to the neck and head. There is a tendency for the rash to spread to the chest, abdomen, arms and legs. The rash may disappear within one week.

Enlarged lymph glands are usually behind the ears, neck and back of head which coincide with areas of initial appearance and spread of the rash. The glands may become painful but unlike the rash may persist for several weeks and may be the first manisfestation of rubella.

Diagnosis of rubella is based on the following:

1. Clinical features (signs and symptoms)
2. salivary test
3. Blood test for antibodies.

Blood test will be positive for IgM antibodies for new cases of rubella and IgG for past history of rubella with antibodies or previous vaccination with the production of antibodies to rubella.

Absence of any of the antibodies excludes rubella and previous successful immunization.

Complications of rubella

This is rare in developed countries where vaccination against rubella (MMR - Mumps, Measles, Rubella) is given usually in childhood as part of routine immunization.

Without maternal protection by immunization either in childhood or adulthood before pregnancy, there is a serious risk of **congenital rubella syndrome (CRS).** This is now rare in the UK as a result of the mass vaccination of mothers and potential mothers.

Congenital rubella syndrome may result in a miscarriage.

The earlier the infection occurs in the course of the pregnancy, the greater the risk to the unborn child as follows:

1. When the infection develops in the first 10 weeks of pregnancy, the risk of CRS rises considerably to 90 per cent culminating in multiple congenital birth defects.
2. When the mother is infected during 11-16 weeks of pregnancy, the risk of congenital birth defects in the baby drops to less than 20 percent.
3. When the mother is infected during 17-20 weeks of pregnancy, CRS becomes quite rare except for occasional cases of deafness.
4. After 20th week of pregnancy, the risk of CRS is virtually nil.

Unfortunately if an unvaccinated mother gets pregnant and becomes infected with rubella virus in the first 20 weeks, immunization or any other treatment will be ineffective in preventing CRS.

As noted above Congenital Rubella Syndrome can cause a number of congenital conditions which may include the following:

1. cataract (opacification of the lens in the eye of the baby)
2. deafness
3. congenital heart disease.
4. microcephaly (congenital small head)

5. slow growth rate
6. damage to the brain, lungs, bone marrow and liver
7. Later on in life, there may be complications of :
8. type 1 diabetes
9. hyperthyroidism (overactive thyroid gland)
10. hypothyroidism (underactive thyroid gland)

Prevention of rubella

Immunization is the safest way to prevent rubella. In the UK, this is given as MMR (Mumps, Measles and Rubella) as part of routine childhood immunization at 12-13 months of age and a booster dose before the child starts school (See immunization programme in chapter one).

Children and adults especially women in the child-bearing age who for some reason did not have the routine immunization are advised to contact their family doctor/GP as immunization may be recommended depending on their history and particular circumstances.

This is particularly applicable to travellers abroad, especially women in the child-bearing age and specifically if travelling to countries where rubella is still prevalent.

People with rubella are infectious for about a week when they are symptomatic before the rash appears and about 4 days after the appearance of rash.

For this reason children who have rubella should :

1. stay off school for the first 4 days after the appearance of rash and if symptomatic a week before then if at all possible that the symptoms are due to rubella and a doctor has been consulted especially if the child is unimmunised.

2. Adults should stay off work for similar reasons.
3. Avoid contact with pregnant women.
4. As rubella is still widespread in certain parts of Africa, Asia and South America, travellers to these areas are advised to have immunization before embarking on their journeys, especially women in the child-bearing age.

Treatment

There is no specific treatment for rubella. Treatment is symptomatic such as controlling fever and pain with paracetamol or ibuprofen.

Children with high fever should be given plenty of oral fluids to prevent dehydration.

SCHISTOSOMIASIS (bilharzia)

This is caused by a parasite flatworm of different species, usually and more commonly Schistosoma haematobium, Schistosoma mansoni and Schistosoma japanicum.

Usually there are no **symtoms** but when they occur, may consist of any of the following:

- abdominal pains
- diarrhoea
- bloody stool
- haematuria (blood in urine)
- pyrexia (fever)
- cough
- joint and muscle pains
- malaise (tiredness, feeling unwell)

These are usually the symptoms of acute scistosomiasis which will depend on the system of the body where the worms or eggs reside or are passing through, which is more often the case in the chronic disease.

The symptoms may improve after a few weeks but treatment is usually advisable as persistence of the worm in the body causes chronic complications.

The **signs and symptoms of chronic disease** may include any of the following symptoms and usually depend on the body system or organs infected as well as the stage of disease :

- There may be itchy red tiny swelling on the skin where the worm burrowed in
- malaise or feeling unwell
- Some people develop fever which may be above 38C.
- There may be abdominal pains.
- Some people may experience joint and muscle pains.

Chronic complications and clinical features may include:

- anaemia usually due to infection of the gastrointestinal tract leading to bleeding which may present as blood in the stool.
- hepatosplenomegaly (enlarged liver and spleen)
- fatigue
- cystitis(inflammation of the urinary bladder)
- dysuria (pain on passing urine)
- haematuria (blood in urine)

Invovement of the heart and lungs may present with :

- cough
- coughing out blood (haempotysis)
- wheezing
- shortness of breath
- Involvement of the CNS(brain and spinal cord) my present with :
- headache
- numbness of the limbs (hands and feet)
- dizziness
- weakness of the limbs
- seizures.

Life history

The parasites are released by fresh water snails and humans become infected through contact with fresh water (rivers, ponds, canals, lakes and reservoirs) which have been contaminated with the parasites.

Transmission occurs when sufferers of the disease contaminate fresh water sources with urine or faeces containing parasite eggs which then hatch in fresh water into tiny lavae and enter freshwater snails. Humans become infected when the larva worms released by freshwater snails penetrate the skin when there is contact with fresh water.

The larva develops into adult worm in the body and lives in blood vessels (usually Schistosoma haematobium). Here the female worm releases eggs which migrate to the bladder or the gastrointestinal tract.

When these eggs pass out through urine or faeces and contaminate fresh water and are taken up by fresh water snails, the cycle continues as noted above.

Some of the eggs are trapped in organs and body tissues and cause immune reactions and the progressive damage to affected organs which become manifest as **chronic disease and complications**. Usually the eggs become trapped in tissues of the liver, spleen, brain, bladder or lungs. The clinical manifestations depend on the organ affected as well as the species of the worm. Without adequate treatment, the worms remain in the body and continue to lay eggs for several years.

Clinical disease is usually caused by inflammatory reactions when the worms lay eggs, secrete proteolytic enzymes that aid the migration to the bladder and intestine to shed the eggs.

Schistosomiasis is **more likely to infect the following**:

1. Farmers who use or come into contact with fresh water
2. fishermen
3. children who like to play in fresh water
4. Poor families who rely on dirty fresh water for livelihood and
5. People who engage in routine agricultural, domestic, occupational and recreational activities in infested fresh water.

The worms may live in the body for years and cause damage to organs such as the liver, kidney, lungs, heart and bladder.

Diagnosis is based on :

1. History of travelling to endemic regions of the world
2. Engaging in activities in fresh water

3. Symptoms and signs of disease
4. Blood test (below)
5. Definitive diagnosis is made by finding eggs of the parasite in urine or stool and by antibodies against the disease in the blood.
6. **Geographical Distribution**

Schistosomiasis is most common in Africa, Asia, South America, the Caribbean, and the Middle East. It is estimated that populations in more than 70 countries and more than 210 million people are affected worldwide with a mortality of 120,000 to 200,000 yearly.

It is one of the listed **neglected tropical diseases by the World Health Organization (WHO)**

Prevention is by:

1. Improving access to clean water
2. Methods to reduce snail population
3. Preventing contact with infested fresh water
4. Travellers to endemic regions should avoid paddling, swimming, bathing or washing in fresh water.Swimming in the sea or chlorinated swimming pool should normally be okay.
5. Travellers and indigens who engage in activities in fresh water, such as crossing a river or pond in endemic areas should wear waterproof trousers and boots.
6. It is possible for the worms to burrow into your mouth if drinking contaminated water. To avoid this, water should be boiled or filtered.
7. Travellers are advised to get treatment at home or seek medical advice on return than rely on local medication which may be fake or substandard.
8. You should not rely on information from local tourist board or hotel. Every fresh water in endemic

regions should be regarded as potentially infected and treated as such.

Treatment.

Treatment with the drug Praziquantel is usually quite effective. A short course is enough to kill the worms.

Steroids may help relieve the symptoms of CNS damage during the acute stage.

Symptomatic treatment of complications should also be carried out.

WHO perspective and distribution of the major forms of schistosomiasis.

The World Health Organization (WHO) estimates that about 258 million people required preventive treatment for schistosomiasis in 2014 and more than 61.6 million were reported to have actually been treated in the same year.

Schistosomiasis transmission has been reported in 78 countries. However, preventive chemotherapy for large scale treatment is only required in 52 endemic countries with moderate to high transmission of schistosomiasis.

Ninety (90) percent of people who require treatment live in Africa. Shistosomiasis is prevalent in tropical and subtropical regions especially in underprivileged or poor communities that lack safe drinking water and basic sanitation.

There are 2 major forms of schistosomiasis-the urogenital and the intestinal and there are 5 main species as follows:

Forms	Species	World Distribution
Urogenital	Schistosoma haematobium	Africa, Middle East, Corsica, France
Intestinal	Schistosoma mansoni	Africa, Middle East, Caribbean, South America (Brazil, Venezuela) (Suriname)
	Schistosoma japonicum	China, Indonesia, Philippines
	Schistosoma mekongi	Lao, Cambodia
	Schistosoma guineensis & Schistosoma intercalatum	Central Africa

TETANUS

Tetanus (lockjaw) is an infection caused by the bacterium, Clostridium tetani, which is commonly found in the soil and manure of animals such as cows and horses.

The bacteria can survive for a long time outside the body.

Dr. Usen Ikidde

Immunization and the proper treatment of wounds and cuts are the best ways of prevention of tetanus.

Tetanus bacteria can get into the body through the following means:

1. Usually through deep wounds containing dirt or foreign bodies
2. Puncture wounds
3. Inconsequential small wounds and cuts
4. Burns
5. Injections by contaminated needles especially by habitual drugs users
6. Eye injury

Signs and symptoms of Tetanus

1. Lockjaw, which is the stiffness and spasms of the jaw muscles which can make opening the mouth difficult.
2. These spasms only last a few minutes at a time but in extreme cases may last up to 3-4 weeks and in a few of those cases, bone fracture could occur.
3. Fever with high temperature of 38 C or more
4. Sweating
5. Difficulty in swallowing due to painful spasm of neck muscles
6. Difficulty in breathing due to the same reason as above
7. Tachycardia (fast heart rate)
8. High blood pressure
9. Irritability
10. Suffocation
11. Incontinence of urine/faeces
12. opisthotonos -arching of back muscles may occur in severe cases.

13. Risus sardonicus- is the appearance of a grin or smile due to muscle spasm of the face.
14. Trismus. The persistent contraction of masseter muscles of the face- around the mouth due to lack of CNS inhibition. It is a feature of generalised Tetanus.

Incubation period

This is the period between exposure and the manisfestation of symptoms. On average this is about 7-14 days but can be shorter or as many as several months.In general, the farther the site of injury from the Central Nervous System-CNS (brain and spinal cord), the longer the incubation period and vice versa.

The bacteria normally produce toxins which become attached to nerves that supply muscle fibres. The stiffness, lockjaw and spasm of muscles are due to the effect of tetanus toxins on these nerves and therefore the muscles, compounded by the overall effect on the CNS which exerts ultimate control.

Types of Clinical tetanus.

There are 4 main types of presentation of tetanus which are based mainly on clinical findings which may relate to age or anatomical region where the infection occurs.

1.**Generalised tetanus** is most common type which involves the whole body and makes up about 80 percent of cases of tetanus.This type tends to present initially with trismus-the persistent contraction of masseter muscles (around the mouth) due to lack of CNS inhibition.Other features of facial muscle spasms also become evident such as lockjaw and risus sardonicus (see above under signs and symptoms).

Generalised tetanus tends to present with a descending pattern from the head downwards.

It follows from this descending pattern that the next anatomical stage is the neck where there is stiffness leading to difficulty in swallowing and rigidity of pectoral muscles. The muscular manisfestations continue downwards where there is stiffness of calf muscles and in severe cases opisthotonos occurs (see above under signs and symptoms).

There are generalised signs and symptoms which may include a high temperature, sweating, raised heart rate and blood pressure.

Muscular spasms may continue for up to a month and recovery may take several months.

Over activity of the sympathetic system is common in severe tetanus and becomes evident with changes in higher than normal blood pressure, fast heart rate, excessive sweating, high temperature and changes in heart rate.

There is normally excessive output of catecholamines (adrenaline and nor-adrenaline) which are hormones that respond to stressful situations such as occur in tetanus. These hormones also cause peripheral vascular constriction. There is increased carbon dioxide output and retention.

These clinical features may be followed by the development of profound hypotension and in severe cases, death occurs within four days.

2. **Tetanus neonatorum** (Tetanus of the newborn)

This is another form of tetanus that occurs in the newborn. It is usually due to failure of the mother to have vaccination against tetanus.The newborn therefore has no passive immunity which would have provided a temporary protection against tetanus as antibodies are able to cross the placenta and provide passive immunity to the newborn until routine active immunization.

The immediate cause is usually due to the use of a non-sterile instrument to cut the umbilical cord during delivery.

Tetanus neonatorum used to be common in developing countries but the situation has generally improved with sustained public health campaign. Secondly the delivery of babies now takes place most often in hospitals or maternity homes where there are trained staff and sterile instruments.

3.**Local tetanus** is the persistent spasm or contraction of the muscles in the same anatomical site of the body where the injury and subsequent tetanus infection occurred.The muscle spasm may take several weeks to subside.Local tetanus is uncommon and usually less serious than generalised tetanus with only about 1 percent mortality. It may often be the prelude to generalised tetanus.

4.**Cephalic tetanus** as the name implies affects only the nerves and muscles of the head.It is rare and usually follows trauma, a contused infected wound and fracture of the skull.It may also follow a dental extraction,eye injury or otitis media. It may arise from injury to other parts of the body but with a cephalic involvement and predominance.

There is usually a facial nerve palsy and other cranial nerves may be involved. The effect may lead to lockjaw.

There is a tendency for cephalic tetanus to progress to generalised tetanus. As a result of the rarity of this form of tetanus, a missed diagnosis is more likely, and therefore carries a high mortality.

WEST NILE VIRUS (WNV)

This viral infection was first isolated from a woman in the West Nile region of Uganda in 1937, hence the name. It was identified in birds in the Nile delta region in 1953.

West Nile virus is transmitted to humans through the bites of infected mosquitoes which themselves become infected when they feed on infected birds which circulate the virus in their blood.

There is no documented evidence of human to human transmission except in utero where maternal-fetal transmission via the placenta is possible.

Signs and symptoms

About 80 percent of infection with WNV is asymptomatic. The remaining 20 percent of infection can cause West Nile fever or severe West Nile disease.

West Nile fever may present with the following symptoms:

- fever
- tiredness
- headache
- nausea
- vomiting

- muscle aches and pains
- skin rash on the trunk
- enlarged lymph nodes

The signs and symptoms of severe disease may include any of the following:

- encephalitis
- meningitis
- high fever
- neck stiffness
- muscle weakness
- convulsions
- tremors
- stupor
- disorientation
- paralysis.

It is estimated that 1in 150 persons infected with WNV will develop the neuroinvasive disease. Whilst the invasive form of the disease can affect any age group, people who are 50 years and over, immunocompromised and transplant patients are at the highest risk of getting the severe form of the disease.

Transmission

West Nile Virus is spread by female culex mosquitoes which transmit the virus during the process of sucking blood from the individual.

The culex mosquito species which transmits the infection varies with geographical location.

In the Eastern United States of America, transmission is by Culex pipiens, whereas in the northern and residential areas, it is by Culex tarsalis, whilst the Culex quinquefascatus are the main vectors in the south east.

In addition to mosquito bites which is the main mode of transmission of the West nile virus, transmission may also occur through the following means:

- blood transfusion
- organ transplant
- intrauterine transmission via maternal placenta to the fetus
- Breast feeding may be responsible for a few cases of transmission.

Geographical Distribution

The largest outbreaks of West Nile Virus have occurred in the following countries and regions :

1. United States of America- imported from Israel and Tunisia
2. Israel
3. Greece
4. Russia
5. Romania
6. Tunisia
7. Parts of Africa
8. Europe
9. Middle East
10. Australia
11. West Asia.

The outbreak WNV in the USA, imported from Israel and Tunisia, underpins the fact that importation and establishment of a vector-borne disease outside a confined geographical area poses a serious danger of global spread.

Complications

Some of the complications have already been alluded to above, but a classification should help to put them in perspective.

The complications may affect the following systems as follows:

1. Gastrointestinal.Nausea, vomiting and diarrhoea may lead to severe dehydration.
2. West Nile encephalitis may present with fever, headache,muscular weakness, flaccid paralysis and altered mental state.
3. West Nile neuroinvasive disease usually follows infection of the central nervous system (brain and spinal cord) resulting in meningitis,encephalitis or WNV poliomyelitis. They may result in muscular weakness.
4. West Nile meningitis may present with fever, headache and neck stiffness.
5. West Nile meningoencephalitis. This is the inflammation of both the brain (encephalitis) and the covering of the brain and spinal cord (meningitis)
6. West Nile poliomyelitis. This usually presents as acute flaccid paralysis with asymmetrical limb weakness or paralysis but with no sensory loss. There may be absence of overt features of infection such as fever and headache.
7. West Nile non-neurological complications which include:

- inflammation of the kidneys (nephritis)
- inflammation of the testicles (orchitis)
- inflammation of the liver (hepatitis)

- inflammation of the pancrease (pancreatitis)
- inflammation of the heart (myocarditis)
- inflammation of the optic nerve (optic neuritis)
- haemorrhagic fever
- irregularity in heart rhythm (arrhythmias or dysrhythmias)
- coagulopathy (disorders of blood clotting)
- skin rash

Diagnosis is based on the following factors:

1. signs and symptoms of WNV
2. endemicity of area of residence
3. Recent visit to endemic region or country
4. If immediately obvious, a recent history of mosquito bite should prove useful. This may begin to ring alarm bell, if there has been a recent visit to endemic region plus any signs and symptoms of West Nile Virus infection above.
5. Armed with the above information, actual confirmation should include the following:

A. (A.) blood test
B. (B.) cerebrospinal fluid (CSF) test obtained by lumbar puncture
C. (C.) Definitive diagnosis is by detection of virus specific antibody IgM and neutralizing antibodies.

Serological testing for WNV is likely to present a problem due to cross reaction with other **flavi viruses** such as dengue and tick-borne encephalitis viruses.

Furthermore WNV testing may not show a positive IgM antibody within the first eight days of infection and a repeat should be carried out later. There may, however, be a positive IgG test which would be indicative of a previous

flavi virus infection but not specific to acute WNV infection.

Under the above circumstances and inorder to confirm WNV infection, sera should be collected and tested both in the acute,chronic or convalescent phases of the illness.

Typical CSF findings show lymphocytes (particular type of white blood cells), elevated protein, reference glucose and lactic levels but no red blood cells (erythrocytes).

In cases of West Nile encephalitis and meningitis,the cerebrospinal fluid also shows substantial increase in one type of white blood cells-the **neutrophils**

Prevention should include the following:

1. The prevention of mosquito bite by:

a. (a)-disposal of tins, cans, tyres, bottles and pools of water to prevent the breeding grounds for mosquitoes.
b. (b)-wearing suitable clothing such as long trousers,long sleeve shirts,socks and hats
c. (c)-the use of mosquito repellent on exposed skin to repel mosquitoes. This could include DEET in concentrations of 30-50% .DEET is usually recommended for adults and children over 2 months of age.
d. Picaridin can also be used and is available in concentrations of 7 and 15 percent.
e. (d)-Mosquito net which is properly tucked under the mattress is recommended for adults and children of all age groups.
f. (e)-Apply Permethrin-containing insect repellents to clothing, mosquito nets, tents and other items.

Permethrin should not be applied directly to the skin. Permethrin has a long lasting effect on clothing and may still be effective even after 5 washings.
- g. (f)-Particular care should be taken during twilight periods (dusk and dawn) when most species of mosquito are more active.
- h. (g)-Staying in air-conditioned rooms may provide additional protection against mosquitoes.

Treatment.

There is no specific treatment for West Nile Virus infection. Treatment should usually be symptomatic and supportive.

All serious cases should be hospitalized and supportive treatment may include intravenous fluids and respiratory support.

MIDDLE EAST RESPIRATORY SYNDROME (MERS)

MERS, also known as camel flu is caused by a corona virus which causes a respiratory infection with varying degrees of severity. MERS is usually more severe in those with other health problems.

MERS, first identified in Saudi Arabia in 2012 was initially confined to the Arabian Peninsula. Since then, spread of this disease has reached several other countries, notably the Republic of Korea where a major outbreak occurred in 2015.

MERS virus is a beta corona virus derived from bats. Antibodies to MERS corona virus have been identified in camels believed to be the main source of spread to humans. The mechanism of spread from camels to humans has not yet been fully elucidated.

Human to human spread is through close contact with an infected person. Such human contacts are therefore more likely to occur in hospitals, within the family and through close social contacts.

As in May 2015, only about a thousand cases have been reported with a mortality of about 40%.

Males are more likely to be infected than females in a ratio of 3.3:1. This preponderance in males may be due to greater and more frequent contact with camels.

The incubation period averages about 5-7 days.

Signs and Symptoms depend on severity, duration and complications of the disease and may include the following:

1. fever
2. cough
3. diarrhoea
4. shortness of breath
5. muscle pain (myalgia)
6. vomiting
7. abdominal pain
8. production of sputum
9. Severe disease or complications may give rise to:
10. severe acute respiratory syndrome
11. pneumonia
12. kidney failure
13. disseminated intravascular coagulation.

Distribution of MERS

Dr. Usen Ikidde

The disease has now spread far and wide outside the confines of the Arabian Peninsula and has been reported or confirmed in the following countries:

1. Saudi Arabia
2. Jordan
3. Germany
4. United Kingdom
5. France
6. Italy
7. Kuwait
8. Omar
9. Qatar
10. Tunisia
11. United Arab Emirates
12. Austria
13. Egypt
14. Greece
15. Iran
16. Lebanon
17. Malasia
18. Netherlands
19. Turkey
20. United States of America
21. Yemen
22. Philippines
23. South Korea
24. Thailand
25. Spain
26. Algeria

Transmission

MERS is a zoonotic virus (a disease that can be passed from animals to humans) Though the specific mechanism of transfer is not fully understood,but it is believed humans become infected through direct or indirect contact with dromedary camels in Middle East Countries.

Strains of Middle East corona virus have been identified in camels in several Middle East countries particularly Saudi Arabia, Oman, Qatar and Egypt.

There appears to be some difficuties in **human to human transmission.** Close contact is necessary to effect this mode of transmission. Such contact often occurs in hospitals or other health institutions where a nurse or a doctor provides regular clinical care to an infected patient. When that occurs without the application and observance of strict hygiene and preventive measures, human transmission is facilitated. For similar reason, family members and other patients in the same ward are also at risk.

If MERS is diagnosed early, isolation of the infected patient remains the best means of preventing spread. Secondly health care workers must be aware and take all necessary preventive measures to prevent getting infected.

Prevention should aim at limiting or actually preventing contact with infected camels. Secondly, prevention of human to human transmission should be by isolation, barrier nursing and by medical personnel taking adequate protective measures to prevent being infected.

Prevention of contact with camels and camel products can be achieved by :

1. Avoidance of physical contact with potentially infected and overtly ill camels.

2. For those who eat camel meat, only properly cooked camel meat should be eaten.
3. Only pasteurized camel milk should be consumed.
4. The practice of drinking camel urine in some Middle East countries where it is considered medicinal, should be discouraged and stopped.
5. The wearing of breathing mask when around camels should be encouraged.
6. The practice of kissing camels by some camel owners should be discouraged and stopped.

The World Health Organization, WHO, further recommends that people who come into contact with MERS suspects should in addition to standard measures, also:

7. Wear medical masks.
8. Wear eye protection (i.e. goggles or face shield).
9. Wear clean, non- sterile, long sleeved gowns and gloves. Some procedures may require sterile gloves and gowns.
10. Perform hand hygiene before and after contact with the patient and his or her surroundings immediately after removal of personal protective equipment (PPE).

For procedures which carry risk of aeronisation, such as intubation, the WHO recommends that care providers also:

11. Wear a particulate respirator and when putting on a disposable particulate respirator, always check the seal.
12. Wear eye protection (i.e. goggles or a face shield).
13. Wear non- sterile long-sleeved gown and gloves (some of these procedures require sterile gloves).

14. Wear an impermeable apron for some procedures with expected high fluid volumes that might penetrate the gown.
15. Perform procedures in an adequately ventilated room;i.e.minimum of 6 to 12 air changes per hour in facilities with a mechanically ventilated room and at least 60 litres/second/patient in facilities with natural ventilation.
16. Limit the number of persons present in the room to the absolute minimum required for the person's care and support.
17. Perform hand hygiene before and after contact with the person and his or her surrounding and after PPE removal.

Treatment.

As at the moment,there is no specific treatment. Current possible treatment are research-oriented and experimental and include the use of interferon, chloroquine, chlorpromazine, loperamide, lopinavir, mycophenolic acid and camostat.

The main treatment is symptomatic- treating the symptoms of the disease like fever, pains,diarrhoea,lung disease etc.

SARS (Severe Acute Respiratory Syndrome)

SARS is caused by SARS corona virus (SARS CoV) which is similar to the virus that causes MERS.

The Corona virus causes infections in animals as well as humans. It is responsible for mild respiratory infections such as the common cold as well as strains of the virus responsible for severe and more serious infections such as SARS.

The more virulent strain of SARS CoV was responsible for 2 major outbreaks in 2002 and 2004-a highly contagious and serious form of pneumonia which fortunately was self-limiting.No further outbreaks have been reported since then.There is no guarantee that there won't be anymore in the future.

The incubation period (time between exposure and onset of symptomatic disease) is about 2-10 days

Symptoms may include the following:

1. A high fever usually over 38C
2. Headache
3. muscle pains (myalgia)
4. Extreme tiredness (fatigue)
5. Loss of appetite (anorexia)
6. Diarrhoea
7. Sore throat
8. Runny nose
9. Chills/rigor

SARS affects mainly the airways and the lungs (the respiratory system).The symptomatic manifestation here may include:

1. Breathing difficulties (dyspnoea)
2. A cough
3. The clinical manisfestation is low oxygen in the blood (hypoxia or hypoxemia).
4. Blood test usually shows low lymphocyte (lymphopenia).

History and Spread of SARS

The first cases of SARS was 2002 in China where the disease originated. From China SARS spread quickly to other parts of the world causing a pandemic. There were no fewer than 8,000 cases and 774 deaths. The infection was fortunately eventually brought under control but not before it had spread to many other Asian countries and many other countries outside Asia including:

1. United Kingdom
2. Canada
3. Taiwan
4. United States
5. Philippines
6. Vietnam
7. Singapore
8. Mongolia
9. Republic of Island
10. Kuwait
11. Romania
12. Russia
13. Spain
14. South Korea
15. Switzerland

Most of the fatalities were in China but there were also some in Canada, Taiwan, Singapore, Vietnam and the Philippines.

SARS CoV is a zoonosis (disease of animals which has mutated to affect humans). It has been isolated in small mammals including bats and civet.

SARS is spread by droplet from person to person by :

Dr. Usen Ikidde

1. Saliva
2. cough
3. sneezing
4. Contact of surfaces by infected person
5. Contaminated hands
6. Through infected person's stool if proper hygiene and washing of hands are not carried out
7. Contact is far more likely to occur through intimate personal contacts with infected people by hospital staff and close relatives at home who care for them.

Prevention

Transmission of SARS virus can be prevented by :

1. covering the mouth properly if coughing
2. covering nose and mouth properly with disposable tissue if sneezing or coughing
3. washing hands properly with soap but especially with alcohol-based hand wash
4. Avoid sharing cup,food, drink,and utensils with infected people.
5. Practise regular cleaning of shared surfaces such as door handles with disinfectant.
6. In suspected and established cases, medical personnel should wear masks,gloves and googgles to prevent being infected by the virus.

Treatment

There is no vaccine and no specific medication to treat the SARS CoV.

1. Suspected cases should be admitted to isolation unit in the hospital.
2. There should be close monitoring.

3. A good clinical history and examination should be carried out.
4. Blood and radiological investigations may be necessary.
5. Supportive treatment should aim at supporting respiration by use of a ventilator.
6. Concomitant bacterial pneumonia warrants antibiotic treatment.
7. Antiviral medications may prove useful and helpful.
8. High dose steroid treatment could help to reduce lung swelling.

ZIKA VIRUS

Zika virus is a vector-borne flavivirus transmitted by the Aedes egypti mosquito-the same mosquito responsible for the transmission of dengue.Flavivirus belongs to the family of viruses responsible for yellow fever, west Nile fever,Japanese encephalitis and dengue fever.

The recent outbreak of Zika virus began in Brazil in April 2015 and spread to other South and Central American countries and the Caribbean.

The name Zika originated from Zika forest in Uganda where the virus was first isolated in 1947. Zika virus then spread to a narrow equatorial region since the 1950s extending from Africa to Asia and then eastwards to the Oceania where there was an outbreak 2013-2014.From there the virus spread to French Polynesia, New Caledonia, the Cook Island and Easter Islands in 2015. The spread then continued to Mexico, Central America,the West Indies and South America where the virus reached epidemic proportions with major congenital health implications especially in Brazil.

Zika virus has been associated with severe brain problems which may result in **microcephaly in newborn babies** and **Guillain-Barre syndrome** in adults.

The Guillain-Barre syndrome is a rare autoimmune disease in which a person's immune system attacks their peripheral nerves.The syndrome tends to affect nerves that control muscle movement and those that transmit sensations of touch, pain and temperature. The syndrome may therefore result in diminished or loss of sensation in limbs or there may be muscle weakness.

This author has seen a picture of a newborn baby in **Nigerian press (United naija, Nairaland Forum 24 January 2016) described as "half human and half donkey".**

A close examination showed that this is a case of microcephaly.It is important to note that this baby also has **a gastroschisis** or **omphalocele** .Basically,this is a congenital herniation of parts of the gut into base of umbilical cord. In short, the baby is born with an open anterior abdominal wall with intestines protruding outside. There are minor differences between the two conditions.The photograph did not make such differentiation possible. Indeed such distinction is immaterial at this stage. The important point here is the congenital abdominal defect in addition to the microcephaly.

This baby was born at the height of Zika virus "pandemic".There are two important questions here:Was there any association with the virus? Secondly, was the congenital abdominal defect in this baby also associated with the virus? This has not been described before and it would add to our understanding and knowledge of the Zika virus if such relationship does, in fact, exist in addition to microcephaly and Guillain-Barre syndrome. This would be of interest to the World Health Organization (WHO) and other reseachers in the field. It is worth noting however that microcephaly is associated with other conditions other than the Zika virus and may include any of the following:

- toxoplasmosis
- chickenpox
- rubella (German measles)
- cytomegalovirus
- drugs
- alcohol
- toxic chemicals
- genetic mutations
- severe malnutrition

Though the current outbreak has not been widely associated with Africa and Asia, but it is worth noting that Zika virus infection had previously been found in Asia, Africa and the Pacific countries.Infact, the name Zika originated from Zika forest in Uganda where the virus was first isolated in 1947.See above.

Development of the virus

Zika virus usually replicates in the midgut of the mosquito and from there migrates to the salivary glands. It takes another 5-10 days for the virus to mature and find its way to the mosquito's saliva which then infects humans when the mosquito bites and inoculates the saliva into human skin. It is thought that the virus then spreads to the lymph nodes and the blood stream. The cycle continues when a mosquito sucks the blood of an infected individual and inoculates the virus into another human.

Signs and symptoms.

Infection with Zika virus is most often asymptomatic and sub clinical. For those who show any symptoms, they are often similar to those of other arboviruses like dengue and include:

1. Fever
2. Headache
3. Muscle and joint pains
4. Malaise
5. Skin rash
6. Conjunctivitis

Geographical Distribution

Zika virus has spread widely to different parts of the world including:

1. Brazil
2. Colombia
3. Dominican Republic
4. Bolivia
5. Barbados
6. Ecuador
7. El Salvador
8. Guatemala
9. French Guiana
10. Guyana
11. Haiti
12. Honduras
13. Martinique
14. Mexico
15. Panama
16. Pueto Rico
17. Paraguay
18. Saint Martin

19. Venezuela
20. Suriname

Transmission

1. , Most cases of transmission of Zika Virus to humans is through the bite of infected Aedes aegypti mosquito and related species.
2. Cases of sexual transmission have also been recorded in the United States,Chile,Argentina,Italy,France and New Zealand.
3. Transmission is usually from male to female and not vice versa.Infected or asymptomatic male could transmit Zika virus to his sexual partner.
4. Zika virus can also be transmitted in utero by infected mother to unborn child via the placenta or during labour.
5. Transmission via blood transfusion has been reported in Brazil.

Prevention

Zika virus vaccine is currently being developed but has not yet reached clinical trial stage.

Prevention is therefore centred around the prevention of mosquito bite by:

1. The disposal of can, tins, broken bottles and pools of water especially in urban and semi-urban areas to prevent the breeding of the Aedes aegypti mosquitoes and similar species.
2. Roof and other gutters should be properly cleared to prevent standing water.

3. Communities that use drums or large containers for water storage should cover them properly.
4. Discard any unused tyres.
5. Leaking pipes which provide a source of standing water should be repaired.
6. Wearing long sleeve shirts, trousers and socks to cover potential areas of mosquito bites
7. Sleeping under mosquito nets which are properly tucked under the mattress
8. Use mosquito repellents.
9. To prevent infection or complications to a newborn baby, women are advised to use contraception or abstinence to prevent pregnancy in endemic areas.
10. Men who have been to endemic areas or have been infected should abstain from sexual activities or use condoms to prevent infecting partners. If they have had suspicion or confirmation of Zika virus infection, this advice should be adhered to for 6 months. If they live or travelled to endemic region but had no symptoms, then this advice should be for at least 8 weeks.
11. Women of child-bearing age should avoid getting pregnant if they have visited endemic areas. It is advisable that they should avoid visiting those areas if at all possible. Where such visit is absolutely necessary, they should adopt all necessary measures to avoid mosquito bites and as no measure provides absolute water-tight protection, they should still avoid getting pregnant shortly before, during, or after such visit for 28 days. This is to obviate possible complications to the baby (See above).

Treatment of Zika virus infection

There is no specific antivirus medication for the treatment of Zika virus infection.

No vaccine has yet been developed and fully tested.

Treatment is normally symptomatic only. Fever and pains are managed with paracetamol (acetaminophen).

It is advisable to avoid NSAID like ibuprofen as there is some risk of bleeding if dengue has not been excluded.

CHAPTER FIVE

SEXUALLY TRANSMITTED DISEASES (STD) -

Now more usually referred to as Sexually Transmitted Infections (STI)

Also called Venereal Diseases (VD).

Sexually transmitted infections (STI) as well as STD are diseases which are transmitted by unprotected sexual intercourse which may be vaginal, anal or oral. Travellers are unlikely to contract any of these infections unless they engage in sexual activities with the local population; some of who might have been exposed to these infections.

Many of these diseases are not confined to any particular regions of the world but are world-wide in distribution and more likely to be found in people with multiple sexual partners or who engage in unprotected sexual activities.

When referred to as Sexually Trasmitted Infections (STI), it usually means that though transmitted sexually, the individual has had no symptoms whereas when referred to as Sexually Transmitted Diseases (STD), it means that symptoms have developed.

Sexually Transmitted Infections (STI) have the propensity to spread easily to other people as there are usually few or no symptoms, at least initially, and therefore, the infected individuals are likely to be unaware that they have been infected and thus withdraw themselves from engaging in sexual intimacy with others.

The original name Venereal disease is derived from the Latin word, venereus, which relates to sexual intercourse or the desire to do so and the word is itself is derived from Venus, the Roman goddess of love which also encompasses prosperity, beauty, fertility and desire.

There are many Sexually Transmitted Infections; some are transmitted almost exclusively by engaging in sexual activities, and others where such activities are not the sole mode of transmission and may actually be acquired more often by other means rather than by sexual encounter. For example HIV can be transmitted via blood, blood products as well as by unprotected sexual intercourse. Scabies is more likely to be transmitted by bodily contact or clothing and bedding rather than by sexual intimacy.

Under such circumstances, sexually transmitted infections and diseases could incorporate or encompass any of the following:

1. Chlamydia
2. Genital Warts
3. Genital Herpes
4. Gonorrhoea
5. Syphilis
6. HIV
7. Trichomoniasis
8. Pubic Lice
9. Scabies
10. Hepatitis B
11. Pelvic Inflammatory Disease
12. Lymphogranuloma Venereum (LGV)
13. Chancroid
14. Molluscum Contagiosum

Dr. Usen Ikidde

CHLAMYDIA

Chlamydia is the most commonly sexually transmitted infection in the UK and the second in the United States.

Transmission is by unprotected sexual activities and especially common in the under 25 and teenagers who make up about 70% of those infected in the UK.

In 2013 there were more than 200,000 people in England who tested positive to Chlamydia and an estimated 1 million in the United States are also infected. World-wide, millions of people are infected.

Chlamydia infection is caused by the bacterium, Chlamydia trachomatis, which is found only in humans and is a major cause of genital and eye disease.

Chlamydia can be transmitted during vaginal, anal or oral sexual activities and can be passed from an infected mother to her baby during childbirth. About 50-75% of infected women are asymptomatic but only have an inflamed cervix.

Men who are infected are more likely to show symptoms than women. They may present with inflammation of the penile urethra and a white discharge which may cause a burning sensation during micturition. Under the circumstance, the infection in men may spread to the epididymis causing epididymitis (inflammation of the area just behind the testicles). In women Chlamydia may spread to the upper genital tract causing a pelvic inflammatory disease which may involve the fallopian tubes and could cause infertility.

For this reason the infection should be promptly treated.Fortunately Chlamydia responds effectively to antibiotic treatment and should not be delayed if the complications and spread to others are to be avoided.

Chlamydia conjunctivitis which is commonly referred to as **trachoma** is a common cause of **blindness** worldwide.Although the incidence appears to be decreasing, it is still a major cause of blindness.The World health Organization estimated that this condition was responsible for 15 and 3.6 percent cases of blindness in 1995 and 2002 respectively.

It is important to recognise the signs and symptoms of Chlamydia in order to make an early diagnosis as delay could cause a number of serious complications.Unfortunately this is more difficult in women where the "Silent Epidemic"may not cause any symptoms at all in about 70-80% of cases and may only be discovered during routine tests.

The signs and symptoms can be classified under the following categories:

1. Genital disease
2. Eye disease
3. Joint disease
4. Disease manifestations in the infant

1.**Genital disease** for the 20-25% of women who may be symptomatic, Chlamydia infection may present with:

- lower abdominal pain
- painful sexual intercourse (dyspareunia)
- vaginal discharge or bleeding
- pain on passing urine (dysuria)

- urgency or frequency of micturition (passing urine)
- fever.
- The symptoms and signs in men are often different from those in women and include:
- whitish discharge from the penis especially in the early hours of the morning on rising from bed
- burning or painful micturition.
- testicular pain which is often more so in the area just behind the testis(the epididymis)
- There may be a swelling and inflammation in this area-epididymitis.

Like in women,spread of this infection to the epididymis may eventually lead to infertility or sterility due to the blockage of the vas-the tube which transmits sperms for fertilization of the female egg-the ovum and since the epididymis provides storage of matured sperms, they could be destroyed due to the widespread inflammation. To prevent this complication, treatment should be instituted at least within 6-8 weeks after exposure to infection; the earlier, the better.

- Spread to the prostate may occur leading to prostatitis and pain.
- Infertility in women is due to an ascending infection from the vulva (vulvitis), vagina (vaginitis), cervix(cervicitis) and the tubes (salpingitis) which may become blocked obstructing the ovum (egg) and the sperm thereby preventing fertilization in the fallopian tube or even if fertilization does occur, the inflammation in the fallopian tube may prevent the fertilized egg from "migration" back to the uterus and thus gets implanted in the tube resulting in ectopic pregnancy.

Ascending infection and inflammation of the fallopian tubes, pelvic lining (peritoneum) and the ovaries leading to pelvic inflammatory disease is additional factor in the causation of infertility in infected women.

Eye Disease

The eye complication of Chlamydia has already been alluded to above, of which blindness is the ultimate and most serious result. Fortunately, the incidence of trachoma has been decreasing and the World Health Organisation aims to eliminate trachoma by 2020.

Child birth through infected mother's genital tract during delivery is not the only means of spread of this infection. It can be spread also from eye to eye by fingers, coughing, sneezing, shared clothes and towels and by eye-seeking flies.

The World Health Ornanisation,WHO, uses **SAFE** strategy (the acronym for **S**urgery of in- growing or in-turned eye lashes,**A** ntibiotics,**F**acial cleanliness, and **E**nvironmental improvement) and the **GET 2020** (**G**lobal **E** limination of **T**rachoma) which aims to eliminate trachoma by 2020.

Joint Disease

One of the symptoms and complications of Chlamydia is reactive arthritis which may manifest in the triad of Reiter's syndrome of arthritis, conjunctivitis and urethritis especially in young men and cervicitis in women. The clinical mnemonic of:

"Can't see,

Dr. Usen Ikidde

"Can't pee and

"Can't climb a tree"

applies to this condition because of its effect on the eye, urinary tract as well as hands and feet being involved in reactive arthritis.

It is estimated that in the United States up to 15000 men develop reactive arthritis due to Chlamydia infection every year and about 5,000 are permanently affected. Whilst reactive arthritis can occur in both sexes, it is more common in men. The triad or just a reactive arthritis and possibly accompanied by the signs and symptoms above may be an important indication to seek medical help.

Disease manifestation in the infant

Chlamydia infected mothers may pass on the infection to the baby during vaginal delivery which may manifest as:

-Conjunctivitis which often occurs **one week** after birth. About 50% of infants of affected mothers will be born with the disease. The timing of conjunctivitis should be contrasted with **conjunctivitis due to gonorrhoea which occurs 2-5 days** and **chemical causes** which usually manifests **a few hours** after birth.

In some cases there may be other manifestations of:

- spontaneous miscarriage (abortion)
- Premature birth
- Conjunctivitis may lead to blindness and
- Unexplained pneumonia affecting the newborn baby.

Screening, Prevention and Treatment

There has been no universally agreed policy on screening. However, there are several recommendations especially in the United States by different Organizations and agencies which include the:

- U.S. Preventive Services Task Force (USPSTF) which recommeds screening women under 25.
- American Academy of Family Physicians recommends screening women 25 years and younger.
- The American College of Physicians recommends screening all at risk.
- The Centre for Disease Control and Prevention recommends the screening of all pregnant women.

This lack of consistency in policy on screening also extends to men where there is also no universally agreed policy.

In the United Kingdom there is an aim but no policy also to :

1. Prevent and control Chlamydia infection through early detection and treatment of asymptomatic infection.
2. Reduce onward transmission to sexual partners.
3. Prevent the consequences of untreated infection.
4. Test at least 25% of the sexually active in the population of under 25 years of age annually.
5. Re-test after treatment.

The infection is quite susceptible to cure by antibiotics such as doxycycline, azithromycin or erythromycin.

Some of these antibiotics are contraindicated or unsuitable during pregnancy; antibiotics such as amoxicillin is not suitable for those with history of penicillin allergy. Erythromycin can be prescribed for those with any history of penicillin allergy.

It is strongly recommended that sexual partners of infected individuals are also treated as otherwise reinfection would occur. Contact tracing of patients who are no longer with their partners should be seriously considered. Both of these principles also apply to many other STIs especially gonorrhoea.

Epidemiology (world distribution of Chlamydia infection)

It is estimated that about 3.1 percent of the world population is infected by sexualy transmitted Chlamydia as at 2010. This is about 215 million people worldwide.

Evidently the infection is more common in women (3.8%) which is likely due to anatomical reasons which is also as a result of the asymptomatic or silent nature of the disease in women than men (about 2.5 %).

It is the second most sexually transmitted infection in the United States and the most common in the United Kingdom.

In the United States it is estimated that there are about 2.8 million new cases a year and 2% of young people are affected.

It is also estimated that about a a quarter of a million cases of epididymitis a year in the United States and nearly half a million of pelvic inflammatory disease cases are due to Chlamydia.

GENITAL WARTS

This is the second most common sexually transmitted infection in England after Chlamydia.Genital warts are caused by the Human Papilloma virus (HPV).

The virus infects the skin through sexual contact which may include vaginal, anal or oral sex and by sharing of sex toys. At the initial stage, they may be quite painless but still capable of causing psychological distress coupled with a sense of uncertainty.

Genital warts present with fleshy growths, skin changes or small bumps around the genital or anal areas. They may be found on the following sites:

In the males

- On the penis
- On the groin
- On the scrotum
- On the thighs
- Inside or around the anus
- In females
- Inside the vagina
- Inside or around the anus
- On the cervix
- Outside the vagina or anus

In both sexes they may also be found on:

- the mouth

- the tongue
- the throat

These are usually due to oral sexual activities with infected person(s).

They may still cause symptoms even in the absence of visibly obvious warts especially in the female where they may cause vaginal discharge, itching, burning sensation or bleeding. The spread or enlargement of genital warts may cause severe discomfort or pain.

Genital warts have a tendency to recur but a few people get only one episode and experience no further problems. When new warts occur, it is difficult to infer whether they are new or due to a recurrence.

Both sexes are affected by genital warts and according to Public Health England there were 73,893 new cases in 2012 diagnosed by Genito-Urinary Medicine clinics(GUM) in England compared to 206,912 cases of Chlamydia during the same period.

It appears that the number of diagnosed genital warts may not tell all the statistical story as people, especially men rarely attend GUM clinics for genital warts.

The strains of HPV that cause cervical cancer are different from those that cause genital warts. There are more than 100 different strains of the virus but only about 30 strains cause warts around the genital skin and specifically 90% of genital warts are caused by only 2 strains of the virus, types 6 and 11.

Prevention and treatment

In the United Kingdom HPV vaccines are offered to all girls aged 12 -13 years old. In a few countries the vaccine are also offered to boys before sexual activities begin. The Mayo clinic Advisory committee on immunization Practice recommends HPV vaccine for girls and boys between ages of 11 and 12.

HPV vaccine called **Gardasil** can protect both men and women against the most common HPV strain responsible for **genital warts and strains that cause cervical cancer.**

Another vaccine called **Cervarix** can protect **against cervical cancer** but not genital warts.

The use of condom can reduce the risk of contracting genital warts but may not completely eliminate that risk.

Topical applications may be used to remove genital warts. These may include:

- Imiquimod (Aldara)
- Podophyllin and Podofilox (Condylox)
- Trichloroacetic acid (TCA)

There may be Genital warts that won't go away . Unsightly warts in particular may cause psychological distress and need to be removed surgically by:

- burning
- freezing
- cutting off the warts
- Laser surgery.

HPV that cause genital warts are also associated with dysplasia-a premalignant state in the cervix. To prevent the development of the premalignant to the cancerous state, it is recommended that women who have had genital warts should have Pap smear test every 3-6 months to monitor changes that may occur in the cervix so that a full malignant change can be averted.

GENITAL HERPIS

This is a common infection caused by herpes simplex virus(HSV) which causes painful blisters on the genitalia and surrounding areas.

Genital herpes is a sexually transmitted infection (STI) which is transmitted by intimate sexual contact. When it affects the mouth area it is referred as **cold sores**.

In the females, it may affect:

- the vulva
- the vagina
- the cervix
- the upper thighs
- the buttocks

In males, it quite often affects:

- the penis
- the scrotum
- the upper thighs
- the buttocks

Symptoms usually appear about 4-7 days after exposure to the virus through sexual acts such as vaginal, anal and oral sexual activities. Kissing may also transmit the virus from one person to another. In fact, this is a common mode of transmission amongst teenagers and young adults.

Genital herpes have a tendency for recurrence but the symptoms tend to be less severe with further episodes which may be due to the acquisition of some immunity to the virus. Recurrence is due to dormancy of the virus in nearby nerves which gets activated especially during stress and periods of ill health. They travel down the nerve roots to the skin and symptoms appear.

The intial infection due to the virus may have the following symptoms:

There may be small blisters which burst leaving red open sores around the affected parts of the body usually the genital area, the upper thighs,rectum or buttocks. There may be:

- vaginal discharge
- blisters and ulcers in the vagina or cervix
- pain on passing urine (dysuria)
- flu-like symptoms
- feeling unwell
- aches and pains

It is possible to pass on the virus to a partner without the infected person showing signs or symtoms.This is the so called **period of asymptomatic or viral shedding**. The risk of doing this is low but tends to be higher during the first year after infection especially with frequent outbreaks of genital herpes infection.

Prevention and Treatment of genital herpes

Like most other sexually transmitted Infections, genital herpes can be prevented by:

- Regular use of condoms
- Use of condoms is useful for all types of sexual activities including vaginal, anal, oral and vulva to vulva contacts.
- It is important not to share sex toys as the virus can be passed on to someone else by so doing.
- Partners should avoid kissing if one partner has cold sores around the mouth.
- Oral sex should be avoided if one partner has cold sores or genital sores.
- Avoid vaginal or anal sex if one partner has genital herpes or infection appears imminent.

Treatment

There are 3 main aims of treatment:

- to relieve pain
- prevent the virus from multiplying and
- to help prevent spread to partner.

Treatment is particularly recommended in the first few days of symptomatic and asymptomatic disease (if known).

Antiviral medications such as Aciclovir, Famiclovir, or Valaciclovir are recommended daily which may be taken up to 5 times a day for 5 days.

For people who have repeated outbreaks several times a year, the antiviral medication can be given for a longer period of time to reduce the number of outbreaks and suppress futher development of genital infections.

Essential Family and Travellers' Health

During pregnancy, one should discuss with the family doctor and the specialist about the advisability of taking antiviral tablets for "a benign condition" like cold sores or genital herpes. Generally, antiviral medication during pregnancy is only advised if the potential benefits outweigh the risks.

Treatment of genital herpes by "off the counter treatment" for cold sores is not recommended as they are generally ineffective. Antibiotics are not recommended also as genital herpes is not caused by bacteria but by a virus.

GONORRHOEA

Gonorrhoea is a sexually transmitted infection.

It is caused by the bacteria Neisseria gonorrhoeae; also called gonococcus.

In the past it was called "the clap."

Gonorrhoea is transmitted by the following methods:

- By unprotected vaginal sexual intercourse
- By Unprotected anal sexual activity
- By sharing sex toys
- During birth, it may infect the baby's eyes.

Gonorrhoea is more likely to infect the urethra of both sexes, the cervix, the rectum and less commonly the eyes and throat.

The infection may be passed to the baby by an infected mother especially through the genital tract during delivery.

Dr. Usen Ikidde

Expectant mothers are strongly advised to have a test and get treated if they are infected.

Symptoms of gonorrhoea-

In Men

- A whitish, yellowish or greenish discharge from the tip of the penis
- Pain on passing urine (dysuria)
- There may be pain in the testicles

In women

- A watery yellowish or greenish vaginal discharge
- Pain on passing urine
- Lower abdominal pain or tenderness
- There may also be intramenstrual bleeding which may sometimes be heavier than normal.

In both sexes -

There may be any of the following:

- If there is infection of the rectum, there may be no signs or symptoms.
- But there may be some discomfort, pain or possibly some discharge.
- Eye infection may present as conjunctivitis, eye pain, swelling or irritation and discharge.
- Throat infection may cause slight pain but this may be absent.

Gonorrhoea infection is quite subtle in women. Often there are no noticeable signs or symptoms at all. In others, the first possible indication may be shown by complications such as pelvic inflammatory disease which with invovement of the fallopian tube could result in infertility.Even when there is a vaginal discharge, distinction from a normal discharge may not be apparent or obvious.Therefore the majority of women are unlikely to be aware that they have the infection. This poses a public health risk of transmission to others who become infected. The bacteria are found in the semen and vaginal fluid of infected individuals who then pass them on during sexual contact with others.

The signs and symptoms may be noticed after 1-14 days especially in men but as explained above, in women there may be no symptoms at all until the infection has spread to other parts of the body leading to complications.

Testing for gonorrhoea infection

It is important to go to your family doctor to ask for a consultation, examination and possibly the test, if you think you have been exposed to the infection especially if:

- You have any of the above signs or symptoms.
- You have recently or in the past had an unprotected sexual intercourse.
- You or your partners have had other sexual partner(s) without any protection.
- Your partner has confided in you that he/she has a sexually transmitted infection (STI).
- You have had a vaginal examination which has been reported as inflamed cervix especially with an unusual discharge.
- It may be necessary to have a routine test if you are pregnant because of the risk of passing the infection to the newborn baby.

The actual **Test** involves the doctor or nurse using a swab to collect a sample of cells from the cervix during a vaginal examination. If there is vaginal discharge, a swab of the vagina may also be carried out.

Sometimes the procedure may be self- administered but such results may be less reliable compared to that carried out by a professional.

The test is not usually painful as only the fluid around the cervix is collected not the actual cervical cells as in a biopsy.

In men a urine sample may usually suffice but where there is copious dicharge from the tip of the penis, this provides another means by taking a swab of the discharge.

The cells may be subjected to immediate microscopic examination but more often it is sent to the laboratory for culture and sensitivity in order to select the right antibiotics to fight the infection.With the development of resistance to some antibiotics, the latter is preferable even if you have to wait for a week or two.

Treatment

Treatment of gonorrhoea infection is by antibiotics which may be by injection, tablets or a combination of both. As explained above, "a culture and sensitivity test" is important to indicate the particular antibiotics which the bacteria are sensitive to, though in some cases treatment can be started before the result of a culture and sensitivity test becomes available. However, this has to be balanced against the possibility of "creating" resistant bacterial organisms and the need for urgency and eradication to prevent complications.

It is also important that your partner is treated as otherwise any treatment could be a waste of time as the infection is likely to recur.To this end, you should tell your partner and previous partners or they can be contacted via contact tracing if acceptable to the parties concerned. This is because contact tracing, though very useful to stem the tide of spread of infection, is actually not compulsory as there is no means of legal enforcement.

As in other sexually transmitted infections, the best way of **preventing infection** is to avoid having multiple partners. It is also important to always use a condom to protect yourself and your partner from sexually transmitted infections. Those who have reasons to suspect that they might be infected (see above) should not hesitate to have a test and receive adequate treatment.

SYPHILIS

Syphilis is transmitted through sexual intercourse with infected person.

It is caused by the spirochete bacterium - Treponema pallidum.

The initial infection presents as infected sore or ulcer and is highly infectious at that stage. Any sexual contact with the sore is likely to transmit the infection which may be during vaginal,anal or oral sexual activities or the use of infected sex toys. Sharing of needle with an infected person may also transmit the infection.

Syphilis can also be transmitted to the unborn baby if the mother is infected. This may be in the form of congenital syphilis if the baby survives. If the unborn baby does not survive it may present as a miscarriage. For this reason, pregnant women are offered routine blood test in the United Kingdom to check for maternal syphilis infection. That is also the case in many other countries. Unfortunately in developing countries where the disease is more prevalent, routine screening for maternal syphilis is not usually the norm.

Syphilis is often referred to as "the great imitator" due to its ability to present in different forms which may easily be confused with other conditions.

The bacteria cannot survive long enough outside the body for transmission to be effected through clothing, sharing cutlery, bathroom or toilet except in exceptional circumstances.

There are 4 stages of the disease with differing symptoms:

1. Primary Syphilis (or stage 1)

During this stage, there is a highly infectious **sore or ulcer on the genital** or around the mouth. This sore or ulcer is referred to as **chancre** which is a firm **painless** skin ulceration or sore and is non-itchy. This is the **stage of high infectivity** when transmission of infection easily occurs through sexual intimacy with an infected person. Sometimes they may be quite unaware of the significance of the chancre which usually appears between 3-90 days after sexual exposure to an infected person.

The chancre may be a single lesion of ulceration with a clean base and sharp edges and less than a centimetre across. Occasionally there are multiples sores or ulcers.

The most common sites are the penis in males and the cervix in the female. The location of the lesion in the female presents a special problem of not being visible to the infected female or to her partner so that infection can easily spread especially if there are multiple partners. In the homosexual male, the lesion is more likely to occur in the anus or rectum which like the female presents the same problem of invisibility and easy transmission and spread of the disease.

There are usually lymph nodes involved which present as inflamed and enlarged lymph nodes especially in the groin.

This stage normally lasts for about 2-6 weeks if untreated and then disappears.

Secondary Syphilis (or stage 2)

Secondary syphilis normally occurs about 3-10 weeks after the primary stage of syphilis. The symptoms of secondary syphilis more often involves the mucous membranes, the skin and lymph nodes. There is usually a reddish- pink rash especially on the palms, sole of the feet and the trunk. The rash may be slightly raised and become infected or may form whitish flat wart-like lesions known as **condyloma latum** found on mucous membranes. The lesions are infested with syphilis bacteria and therefore **very infectious** if in close contact with other people in susceptible areas. Such transmission is more likely to occur if the lesions occur in the female genitalia or the anus.

Other symptoms also occur and in totality the following symptoms and signs may be encountered in secondary syphilis:

- rash
- fever
- malaise

- hair loss
- headache
- weight loss
- There may also be:
- kidney disease
- inflammation of the liver
- joint inflammation
- optic neuritis (inflammation of the optic nerve)
- uveitis (inflammation of the uveal tract in the eye)

These symtoms and signs tend to disappear after about about 4-6 weeks; however in about a quarter of those infected, there may be recurrence of symptoms. Many of those who present with secondary syphilis, were either not actually aware of when they had symptoms of primary syphilis or attached no significance to the lesions.

The Latent stage

Stage 2 or secondary syphilis usually disappears after a few weeks when there are no symptoms. The only proof that the individual had been infected in the past is a positive blood test or a history of untreated syphilis. This stage without symptoms is the latent or hidden phase of syphilis. The early stage of latent syphilis is usually regarded as 1-2 years after the secondary stage and the late latent syphilis after 2 years. The possibility of a relapse of symptoms is more likely to occur in the early latent period which is also more contagious than the late latent period. Latent stage may last for several years.

Tertiary Syphilis (or stage 3)

After varying period of about 3-20 years after the initial infection, tertiary syphilis and the most dangerous stage develops and is usually divided into 3 forms:

- Gummatous syphilis
- The late neurosyphilis
- Cardiovascular syphilis

About one third of untreated cases of syphilis develop tertiary syphilis. Though the most dangerous in terms of the effect it has on sufferers but tertiary syphilis is **not infectious**.

Gummatous Syphilis which occurs after several years of untreated disease is characterised by the formation of gummas. Gummas are rounded inflammatory soft and tumour-like structures which typically affect the skin, bones and the liver.

The late **neurosyphilis** affects the central nervous system. It may be asymptomatic or show signs and symptoms which may include the following:

- meningitis
- general paresis
- tabes dorsalis-manifests as lightening pains in the lower limbs or/and poor balance.

At the late stage it may present with clinical features of neurovascular involvement and may include:

- apathy
- fits (seizures)
- dementia
- tabes dorsalis
- Argyl Robertson pupil characterised by bilateral small pupils(of the eye) in which constriction is evident on focusing on near objects but no constriction to exposure to bright light.

Cardiovascular syphylis may take several years 10-30 after initial infection. The most common complication here is inflammation of the aorta (**syphilitic aortitis**) which weakens the wall of the aorta and may result in **aneurysm (**dilatation of the wall of the blood vessel).An aneurysm may be complicated by pressure on neighbouring structures, leakage and eventually bursting with cardiovascular collapse and death.

Congenital Syphilis

When a mother is infected with syphilis, the unborn child could suffer a number of detriments and when born, there could be a number of life threatening conditions and deformities which may include any of the following:

- miscarriage (mother)
- stillbirth
- prematurity
- neonatal death
- seizures
- fever
- rashes .
- rhinitis (snuffles) with T. pallidum bacteria which are infectious.

These symptoms may be unnoticed passing through latent syphilis stage but later manifesting with damage or deformities to:

- eyes- inflammation of the cornea (interstitial keratitis)
- ears- deafness
- bones- frontal bossing- prominence of the brow ridge
- teeth -may be blunted (Hutchinson's teeth)

- brain- may lead to psudoparalysis

There may be deformities and other signs including:

- Saddle nose (collapse of the bony part of the nose)
- Deformities of the lower limb and other bones
- Short maxilla
- Deformities of the hard palate
- Protruding Mandible
- Swollen knees
- Anaemia
- Jaundice
- Enlarged Liver (Hepatomegaly)
- Enlarged spleen (splenomegaly)
- Enlarged lymph nodes(Lymphadenopathy).

Prevention and Treatment of Syphilis

Syphilis can be prevented by the following measures:

- Avoiding sexual contact with people with unknown disease status
- Avoiding sexual activities with multiple partners
- Use of male or female condoms
- Avoid oral contact with partner's genitals or anyone whose disease status is unknown or suspicious.
- Avoid sharing sex toys.
- Drug users and addicts should avoid sharing needles.
- If your partner has a history of other sexually transmitted infections or is a new partner with suspicious history,you should have him/her tested and treated accordingly before any sexual contact.
- Those people with signs and symptoms or history of exposure should be tested as soon as possible and get effective treatment if infected.There should

be no sexual contact until they have been cured and declared disease free.
- Avoid touching the sores and ulcers of syphilis as infection can be transmitted without sexual contact.
- Avoid kissing an infected partner or person.
- All mothers should be screened for syphilis during antenatal clinic and early effective treatment instituted, if infected, to prevent exposure of the unborn and newborn child to maternal infection.
- Where no screening had been carried out and maternal infection is discovered late in pregnancy, it is still better to offer treatment than not treating at all.

In cases where maternal screening was not carried out, the newborn baby should be tested and treated accordingly.

Early treatment of infected people should be the norm. Penicillin is the antibiotic of choice but your doctor or specialist would decide the best treatment for individuals with history of allergy to penicillin or resistance.

Other antibiotics in use include Doxycycline or Tetracycline but are not recommended during pregnancy due to risk of birth defects.

Ceftriaxone is another effective alternative to penicillin.

Those undergoing treatment are advised to avoid sexual contact with partners until treatment has been completed, all sores or ulcers have healed and have been declared disease-free by the specialist who treated them.

HUMAN IMMUNODEFFICIENCY VIRUS (HIV)

HIV or Human immunodeficiency virus is a viral infection that attacks the immune system, weakens it and thus reducing its ability to fight infections and disease.

HIV is caused by a retrovirus. which can progress to AIDS (acquired immune deficiency syndrome) when the progressive failure of the immune system allows life-threatening opportunistic infections and specific types of cancers to thrive. There is no cure for HIV but medications are now available which stop the progression of the disease. When this occurs, the individual can live an almost normal life despite the infection in the system.

HIV is transmitted by certain body fluids which include the following:

1. Blood
2. Semen
3. Vaginal fluid
4. Pre-ejaculate fluid and
5. Breast milk of an infected mother.

The most common mode of transmission are the following:

- Having unprotected vaginal sexual intercourse
- Having unprotected anal intercourse
- By sharing needles usually by drug abusers/ addicts
- By HIV positive mother transferring infection to either the unborn baby during pregnancy, delivery or by breast feeding.
- By blood transfusion of whole blood or blood products - now rare.

Dr. Usen Ikidde

Some vital cells in the human immune system are infected by HIV virus and these include some helper T cells especially those called CD4+ T cells, macrophages and dendritic cells. Thus HIV infection lowers the level of CD4+ T cells. HIV viruses exercise their destructive functions by a number of mechanisms including the direct viral killing of infected cells and the killing of infected CD4+ T cells which are carried out by CD8 cytotoxic lymphocytes that are able to recognise infected cells. The progressive decline of CD4 +T cells continue until a critical level is reached when the cell- mediated immunity is entirely lost and susceptibility to opportunistic infection reaches a crescendo and the body's defence mechanism is no longer capable of fighting off such infection.

There are two types of HIV which are characterized as HIV-1 and HIV-2. The first type of the virus discovered was HI-1 which is more virulent and infective and causes most of the HIV infections world-wide.

HIV -2 on the other hand has a lower infectivity and fewer of those exposed to this type will be infected per exposure. HIV- 2 is mostly found in West Africa and this may explain the lower prevalence of HIV in this region compared to East,Central and South Africa.

History of HIV and AIDS

Clinically proven, laboratory tested and confirmed AIDS and HIV as we know it today was first observed in the United States of America in 1981amongst injecting drug users and gay men (homosexual males) with no known cause of impairment of immunity who developed a rare form of opportunistic infection - pneumonia with Pneumocystis carinii.

Some other homosexual men developed a rare type of skin cancer called Kaposi's sarcoma.

1. No name or origin of this new disease was found, and so the name **Gay-Related Immune Deficiency** (**GRID**)was coined.
2. Soon after this, it was found that there were some groups who were more often infected and these included the following:

Homosexuals = H

Heroin users = H

Haemophiliacs = H

Haitians = H

For this reason the name **4H** was coined.

3. Later it was discovered that HIV and AIDS infected Human T - Lymphocyte cells and the name was changed to Human T- Lymphotropic virus.

=**HTLV**

4. The evolution in HIV and attempts to find the most suitable name to take into account all circumstances of the disease still continued. The association of HIV and AIDS with enlarged lymph glands led to the formation of another name to embrace this finding and so the name **Lymphadenopathy - Associated Virus** = **LAV** was coined.
5. The end of this journey was in sight and a new name that would embrace the most important pathological features of this disease which is the

immune deficiency that it causes to humans was coined, and so the name **Human Immune - deficiency Virus** eventually emerged and so **<u>HIV</u>** became the most acceptable name in 1986.

There were no specific, clinical, immunoassay tests, Enzyme -linked immunosorbent assay (ELISA), nucleic acid testing (viral RNA or proviral DNA amplification method) which confirmed HIV prior to the 1981 when this disease was first discovered in the United States.

Attempts to pin the origin of HIV or AIDS as having originated from certain other areas of the world are therefore purely speculative and clearly lacks scientific proof, clinical acumen and argument to support it.

There is a school of thought but no definitive proof that the 2 subtypes of HIV, - HIV-1 and HIV-2 are believed to have originated in non-human species- primates in West Central Africa and thought to have transferred to humans (zoonosis) in early 20th century. There is absolutely no confirmed scientific basis for this belief. It is a theory and like all theories, it lacks proof, sound scientific basis or evidence. In short, it is speculative, conjectural and presumptive.

There is absolutely no proof for this assumption that there was an unusual zoonosis in which the viral infection completely abandoned the initial host- primates, and chose to settle only in humans. There appears here to be a deliberate ploy to pin this disease to Africa and not the United States where this infection was first discovered, when scientific and clinical evidence are clearly lacking.

The earliest documented case dates back to Belgian Congo in 1959 when there were no tests to confirm that this was HIV infection. Such speculation is therefore by extrapolation. There are many infections- bacterial and viral which mimic HIV and unless the laboratory and clinical pictures are in consonance and proven by today's standards or even half today's standards then the assumption clearly fails to measure up.

The proven case shows that the virus was already present in the United States as early as the mid to late 1950s where a 16 year old male presented with symptoms of HIV in 1966 and died 3 years later having had the disease since the mid 50s . This suggests that AIDS was present in the United States some 4-5 years before the 1959 unconfirmed case in Belgian Congo.What is surprising is how the infection would have disappeared for so many years until its re-emergence and again in the US in 1981. Were these 2 cases in Belgian Congo and the US really due to HIV ?

It is difficult for this author to see how Africa with its poor medical services could contain an infection with endemic and pandemic potentials and dimensions for more than 25 years as no other cases were found or reported. It is therefore almost incredible to believe that the 1959 case was really due to HIV. Did HIV go into hibernation after the 1959 single incident.? It is well known that in Africa blood and blood products were not routinely screened for HIV until lately. There was also no significant change in sexual life style either in the United States or Africa. The use of condoms is a recent introduction to contain the virus and other STIs and also for contraception.

Symptoms of HIV infection

HIV usually takes about 2-6 weeks after exposure to produce symptoms of infection which may include some or all of the following:

.Flu-like illness, when seroconversion takes place and may last for 1-2 weeks or even longer as the immune system resists or tries to fight off the infection.

- Fever
- Sorethroat
- Rashes
- Joint pains
- Muscle pains
- Tiredness
- Enlarged lymph nodes

.After the disappearnce of these initial symptoms, there is an asymptomatic period that could last for several years which is unrecognisable but during which the virus is still active and progressively continue to damage the immune system.

The asymptomatic period could last for up to ten years or more during which time the infected individual may feel well and appears well.

After the asymptomatic period and the immune system has been severely damaged, other symptoms may include the following:

- Night sweats
- Weight loss
- Chronic diarrhoea
- Recurrent infections
- Life-threatening illnesses

Early treatment may help prevent these symptoms.

Screening

Routine antenatal screening should be carried out during antenatal period. If HIV infection is untreated, it could be passed on to the unborn child during pregnancy via the placenta, during delivery and through breast feeding.

HIV Test

It is important to get tested when one has been exposed to HIV or develops any of the symptoms above. It is also important to realise that it takes about **a month** after the infection for enough antigens and antibodies to build up in the blood in order to obtain a reliable positive test.

However, it is still necessary to report and have a test booked even when there are no symptoms. After about a month the test should be carried out to confirm the result.

A simple HIV test would usually check for the presence of antigens and antibodies in the blood. It is now possible also to test for HIV using your saliva or a pin prick to the finger which only utilises a tiny blood-spot.

HIV tests are usually carried out with an informed consent of the individual concerned as there are implications which could affect different aspects of your life including job and employability. For similar reasons, access to the results is also restricted.

It is usual to get back the result within a week though some clinics offer rapid testing facilities when results are available within half and hour.In all cases, a positive result should be repeated for a confirmation and a negative result, if in doubt, should also be repeated.

Dr. Usen Ikidde

Testing can be carried out by some general practitioners, a genitourinary Medicine (GUM) clinic, rapid testing clinics, private clinics, and some contraception clinics.

The test for HIV-1 is usually by an enzyme linked immunosorbent assay **(ELISA)** which detects antibodies to the virus. A specimen which is non reactive to this test is regarded as HIV negative unless there is a new exposure to the virus. When a specimen has reacted to ELISA test, it**requires retesting in duplicate**.When the result of either duplicate is reactive, the result may then be **reported as repeatedly reactive** and a**confirmatory test** would then be required with a more specific supplemental test by say,**Western blot test** or the immunofluorescence assay **(IFA).**

It is only after the whole process above has been carried out that the patient can be regarded as HIV positive.

There are also less commonly used tests- the nuclei acid testing which involves the viral RNA or the proviral DNA amplification methods.

The accuracy of HIV testing has been greatly enhanced by these modern methods and the overall accuracy is now estimated to be more than 99% and the chance of a false positive with the standard 2 step method is estimated to be very small especially in a low risk population.

In summary, and in order to achieve accuracy, HIV testing should start with an immunoassy combination test for HIV-1 and HIV-2 antibodies and antigen. A negative result would usually rule out HIV whilst a positive result would require a follow up by an HIV-1/HIV-2 antibody differentiation immunoassay to find out which of the 2 HIV types is present or whether the 2 types are present in the same sample.

Prevention and Treatment of HIV

The most important ways of preventing HIV are the following:

- Abstinence especially with unknown or untested partner
- The use of condoms
- Both new partners should be tested if need be before engaging in sexual intimacy.
- Avoidance of multiple partners
- People with other sexually transmitted infections are more likely to be infected with HIV and should therefore opt for testing before engaging in sexual activities with a new partner.
- Sexual contact should be avoided if there are ulcers on the genitals which may suggest STI such as syphilis.
- When unsure, take the safe and avoidance option.
- In endemic areas, circumcision has been shown to reduce infection and should be seriously considered.
- Routine HIV testing should be carried out for all pregnant mothers during antenatal clinic.
- Effective and early treatment of infected mothers should be the norm.
- Mothers should not breast feed their babies if they are HIV positive.

Treatment of HIV

HIV treatment should be commenced in people who have been confirmed as HIV positive and have had regular blood tests to monitor the progress of the infection.

This usually involves monitoring the amount of virus in the blood as determined by the level of CD4 +T lymphocyte cells in the blood which are important in the fight against infection.

Generally, treatment should be commenced when the CD4 cell count falls towards or below 350 mark irrespective of the presence or absence of symptoms. Usually the specialist determines when to start treatment by taking other parameters such as the general health and other diseases into consideration not just the CD4 levels. For patients who have conditions such as hepatitis B or C, tuberculosis, kidney or brain disease or are on radiotherapy or chemotherapy, treatment should be started at a much higher CD4 level such as when there is a fall just below 500.

HIV is treated with antiretroviral (ARV)combination medication which works by stopping the replication of the virus in the body and helps the immune system to repair itself and prevent further damage.

The virus has the propensity to adapt and become resistant to medication. The best solution to this is the use of combination medication. Some have actually been combined into one pill which makes it easier to take. This is the "fixed dose combination".

There is no cure for HIV and the medications will usually need to be taken for life and on a regular basis unless there is a breakthrough in research with the development of a vaccine. Skipping or forgetting to take the pills may reduce effectiveness and lead to resistance.

Drug reactions, interactions and resistance should be avoided by making sure that other medications taken are reported to the doctor and the antiretroviral medications are taken daily and regularly as prescribed.

TRICHOMONIASIS

This is a common sexually transmitted infection caused by a tiny flagellated parasite called **Trichomonas vaginalis**.

More than half of infected people -both men and women, have no symptoms of the disease. When symptoms are apparent, they are usually evident about four weeks or less after exposure to the infection. This infection is more common in women than men and because of the passage of time older women are more likely to have been infected (**prevalence-**old prevailing cases) than younger ones. However the **incidence (**new cases) is higher in younger than older women which may be due to more frequent exposure to infection.

The disease is transmitted by having unprotected vaginal intercourse, or female-female vaginal or vulval intimacy.

Trichomoniasis in women usually affects the vagina, vulva and/ or the urethra and the following **symptoms** may be experienced:

- Soreness.
- Itching may be a prominent feature.
- A greenish,-yellow, frothy or watery vaginal discharge
- The discharge is usually more than the usual discharge and may have an unpleasant fishy smell.
- There may be unusual pain on passing urine or during sexual intimacy.
- There may be some lower abdominal pains.

In men the following parts may be affected:

- Urethra

- The prostate
- The foreskin
- The urethral opening

The following symtoms may be experienced by men:

- Painful micturition (passing urine)
- Painful ejaculation
- Whitish discharge from the penis
- There may be redness, inflammation and soreness around the tip of the penis and the foreskin.

Diagnosis

Diagnosis of Trichomonas vaginalis infection should be based on the following:

1. Clinical features -symptoms and signs which indicate infection.
2. Swab from the vagina, urethra, cervix or the penis, which are then subjected to saline microscopy. This has a low sensitivity.
3. Culture of the organisms
4. Nuclei Acid Sensitivity amplification Test (NAAT). This is the most sensitive test.

Prevention

1. Use of condoms may help to prevent the spread of Trichomoniasis.
2. Diagnosis and treatment of those who are symptomatic
3. Currently there are no official screening programmes. This should be encouraged and implemented.

4. There should be tracing of sexual partners and treatment to prevent further spread.
5. Recurrence of this infection is common and the contact tracing of current and previous partners should be given due consideration.

Treatment

Metronidazole (Flagyl) is the antibiotic of choice but requires caution in early pregnancy and specialist opinion should be sought.

A small percentage, about 5% are resistant to Metronidazole and this may account for recurrence in some patients.

Sexual partners should be treated even if asymptomatic, otherwise recurrence is likely to occur.

Trichomoniasis tends to persist in women but spontaneous resolution typically occurs in men.

Complications

Infection with Trichomonas vaginalis is more likely to be associated with other STIs especially HIV.

Low birth weight and premature babies are more common if the mother is infected.

In males, infection may be complicated by prostatitis and urethritis and the former may lead to prostate cancer.

Dr. Usen Ikidde

PUBIC LICE (Pediculosis pubis or Phthirus)

Pubic or crab lice are regarded as sexually transmitted infection because they usually infect people who come into close sexual contact with each other. For this reason adults are more easily affected than children.Transmission can also occur through non- sexual contacts especially through the sharing of towels, clothing, and beds by family members.Non-sexual transmission are not as common, as pubic lice can only survive for a short period of time outside the warmth and humidity of the human body.

Pubic lice (Phthirus pubis) can take many weeks before the manifestation of symptoms which include:

- itching especially in the skin of pubic hair area: this could be quite intense.
- irritation and inflammation caused by scratching
- There may be blood on underwear caused by scratching.
- There may be blue coloured spots on the affected area due to bites by pubic lice.

The itching is attributable to an allergy due to lice saliva rather than a bite by the pubic lice.

The itching is usually worse at night which is when the lice are more active and deposit more saliva on the affected part of the body.

Pubic lice are tiny and difficult to see clearly with the naked eye;they are about 2mm long and are dusky red or yellowish grey in colour.

They have 6 unequal legs, 2 of the legs being larger than the others, claw-like and capable of grasping and hanging onto hairs.

Pubic lice are different from the lice that infest the head hair and can live on the hairs on other parts of the body such as the armpit, chest, body hair, beards, moustache and eyelashes.

Pubic lice lay eggs(nits) which are contained in sacs that are firmly stuck to hairs. They are pale brownish in colour and when the eggs hatch they leave behind whitish empty sacs.

Prevention

- Prevent sexual and close contact with an infected person.
- Early treatment to prevent transmission to a partner and close family members.
- Avoid sharing towels and other items of clothing.
- Regular laundry of personal items of clothing of infected person including underwear, bedclothes and towels.

Treatment

Topical agents such as permethrin or pyrethrins with piperonyl peroxide are quite effective. Anther agent such as Lindane, which forms the second line treatment is limited by its toxicity especially during pregnancy, lactation, people with extensive dermatitis and children under 2 years of age.

Dr. Usen Ikidde

SCABIES

This is a contagious skin disease.

It is caused by tiny mites(Sarcoptes scabiei) that burrow into the skin. Scabies are usually transmtted through sexual or skin to skin contact and from bedding, towels and clothing. Scabies prefer warm places, such as irregular or unexposed parts of the body like skin folds, under finger nails, between fingers, breast creases and buttocks.

The main symtoms of scabies are **itching** and **rash.**

The itching is usually intense and is worse at night due to warmth and less distraction. The itching is mostly in the areas of the body where the mites have burrowed into.

It may take upwards of 4-6 weeks after exposure for itching to start which is the period of time it takes the body to react to the droppings which cause the itching.

For those who have had scabies before , the itching could start within 24-36 hours as the immune system had already been primed to recognise and respond to scabies infection.

The rashes are small red spots. Scratching is common due to the intense itching and leads to the formation of crusty sores which may become infected.

The burrows made by the mites may be found virtually anywhere on the body but are more likey to be found in the following places in adults:

- The wrist
- The palms of the hand
- Skin folds between fingers or toes

- Soles and sides of the feet
- The elbows
- Area of the nipple especially in women
- Genital area especially in men

The rash caused by the mites tends to affect almost the whole body except the head but the following areas are particularly prone:

- The groin
- The female genital area
- The underarm area (armpit)
- around the waist
- Below the area of the lower buttocks
- Lower legs
- Around the ankle
- The knees
- Inside of the elbow region
- The area around the shoulder blades
- The sole of the feet
- Men may have one or more very itchy and lumpy spots on the skin of the penis and/ or scrotum.
- In the immunocompromised people, the elderly and the young, there may be rashes on the head and neck.
- Infants and the young tend to have burrow marks in unusual places compared to the adult and these may include:
- the head
- the face
- the scalp
- the neck
- soles of the feet
- the palms of the hand

There is a tendency for infection of the burrows or a concomitant bacterial infection to occur on the palms and soles of the feet with blisters and possibly pustules in infants and those people with low immunity.

Prevention

Scabies infestation can be prevented by paying attention to the following:

- Attention to personal hygiene
- Avoiding sexual intimacy with affected individuals.
- Mass treatment programmes by using topical applications.See below
- Avoid sharing personal items of clothing especially towels, underwear and bedding.
- Frequent laundry of bedding, underwear and towels
- Contact tracing and treatment even if they exhibit no signs and symptoms.
- The mites can survive for 2-3 days without a host; therefore cleanliness and frequent washing and laundry of items of clothing above should be the norm especially in the case of crusted scabies.

Treatment of scabies will only succeed if it invovoles the entire household and those who have had prolonged physical or sexual contact with affected individuals.

Itching can be controlled with antihistamine, some of which may also cause drowsiness and allow for sleep to prevent excessive scatching.

The actual and effective treatment of scabies is by application of **Permithrin** before bedtime and left for about 8-14 hours before washing it off in the morning.It is important to apply to the whole body and not just the affected areas as untreated areas may provide safety for the mites to escape to and survive. Only one application is sufficient to kill the mites and eggs. However, some doctors recommend a second treatment 3-7 days later as a precautionary measure to ensure effectiveness. Crusted scabies may also require multiple treatments with Permithrin or occasionally in difficult cases supplemented with the oral agent **Ivermectin** which can be useful in crusted scabies. See below. The latter is not recommended for children under 6 years of age.

There are also other preparations which have been shown to be useful or effective. These include:

- Benzyl benzoate
- Crotamiton
- Malathion
- Sulfur preparations
- Lindane, though effective, is limited by concerns over potential neurotoxicity.

Scabies Outbreak

Scabies is a global problem but is widespread in densely populated areas of the world with limited resources and medical care.

It is more common in:

- Africa
- India
- Southeast Asian countries
- South and Central America.
- Central and northern Australia
- The Caribbean

Scabies outbreak occurs also in developed countries particularly where there are congregations of people such as schools, families with overcrowding, care homes and nurseries.

In the United Kingdom, outbreaks tend to occur in the winter months when there is a tendency to spend more time at home and thus more social and bodily contacts.

Complications of Scabies infection

Generally if diagnosed and treated in time, scabies should not lead to life -threatening conditions. However the following problems may arise due to poorly managed or untreated scabies:

1. Infection- repeated itching and scratching may lead to infection of the skin and worse still may result in:
2. Impetigo- a more serious form of skin infection

3.**Crusted scabies.**(Norwegian scabies) This is a serious form of scabies where there is an overwhelming infestation with scabies mites in thousands or millions. This is usually seen in the immuno-compromised people or may follow a skin reaction and could affect all parts of the body-the head, trunk, neck, nails and scalp.

Unfortunately the rash associated with crusted scabies doesn't itch thus making a diagnosis difficult and may be mistaken for psoriasis.

Crusted Scabies tends to affect :

- the very young
- pregnant women

- people with neurological (brain) disorders such as Parkinson's disease
- people with Down's syndrome
- the elderly
- people with weakened immune systems such as HIV and AIDS
- people on chemotherapy
- those people on steroids.

HEPATITIS B VIRUS

This is an infectious disease of the liver caused by hepatitis B virus. It may be acute or progress to chronic disease. Many of those infected do not experience any symptoms during the initial disease or may simply fail to notice it due to the mild nature of the symptoms in some individuals.

Hepatitis B is only one of the five known hepatitis viruses A,B, C, D, E which are infective to man and can be transmitted generally in the same manner between individuals and spread to the liver and so the name, "hepatitis" (inflammation of the liver).

For those who experience symptoms, it may only last for a few weeks and may consists of any of the following:

- Loss of appetite
- Nausea
- Body aches and pains
- Vomiting
- Low grade fever
- Jaundice (yellowness of the eyes)
- Tiredness
- Abdominal pains
- Dark urine

- Itching of the skin

Hepatitis B may be transmitted by the following routes to people at risk who should be vaccinated:

- Blood transfusion via unscreened blood
- Sexual intercourse (vaginal secretion, semen)
- Maternal transmission to baby during delivery
- Via infected needles by intravenous drug users
- Health Care workers by needle stick injury at work
- Dialysis
- Living with infected person may increase the risk due to exposure or sexual intimacy.
- Living in an institution may increase the risk due to exposure -above.
- Tattooing with infected instruments
- People with liver disease have increased risk and should be vaccinated.
- People with chronic kidney disease have increased risk and should be vaccinated.
- Acupuncture with infected needles should be avoided. Users of such facilities should be vaccinated.
- Families who adopt children from high risk regions should be vaccinated.
- Male and female sex workers should be vaccinated against the virus.
- Prisoners and people in similar institutions should be vaccinated as there is increased risk due to exposure.
- Visits to endemic areas may increase the likelihood of contracting the disease especially if there is sexual intimacy with the local population, intravenous drug use or exposure to infected blood and blood products.

It could take as long as 30-180 days for symptoms to manifest after exposure.

Complications

Those who are infected at birth have a 90% chance of developing chronic disease but after the age of 5 there is only about 10% chance. The main complications of chronic disease are:

- Cirrhosis of the liver
- Cancer of the liver
- Both chronic conditions may lead to death.

Risk of Maternal Transmission of Hepatitis B to the baby

There are many people who are infected with hepatitis B but do not show any signs or symptoms but are carriers and can transmit the infection to others.

This is particularly important during delivery when maternal transfer can and does occur.

In the UK as in many other countries, pregnant women are routinely tested for hepatitis B during their visits to the antenatal clinic. Those with positive results are immunized accordingly to prevent the transfer to the baby at birth.

Babies at birth who are considered to be at risk are immunized in the first 24 hours, followed by 2 more doses at one and two months and a booster at 12 months. Antibody immunoglobulin may also be judged necessary and given to the baby at birth. This is particularly important if the infection in the mother was not detected in time and the baby is at risk.

Immunization at birth is about 90-95 percent effective and the goal is to prevent the development of chronic hepatitis B infection later in life as 90 % of babies infected at birth develop chronic hepatitis whilst only about 10% of those infected after 5 years of age progress to the chronic disease.

This author also wishes to draw attention to the fact that in addition to other modes of transmission, as for hepatitis B, Hepatitis **C is also sexually transmitted** as well as maternal transmission during delivery though the risk is less than with hepatitis B.

Unfortunately there is no effective immunization currently to prevent Hepatitis C. Tests are available to detect the infection either in the adult or baby who should then be referred to the specialist.

Prevention of Hepatitis B

1. Since 1982, effective immunisation has been developed to combat this virus. The World Health Organization (WHO) recommends vaccination in the first 24 hours of life. This is followed by 2 or 3 more doses in order to achieve the full effect. As stated above the vaccine is 90-95 percent effective if given in this manner.
2. All blood and blood products should be screened for hepatitis B before transfusion.
3. It is recommended that condoms be used for sexual intimacy to prevent infection with the virus.
4. Screening for the virus should be carried out for those who have not been vaccinated, intravenous drug users, those with HIV, homosexual males and

those who share the same living accommodation with an infected person.
5. Healthcare workers who may come into contact with the virus should be vaccinated.
6. Pregnant women should be offered screening for the virus and vaccinated if the test is positive and the babies vaccinated as stated above.

Treatment of Hepatitis B.

It must be emphasized that prevention is better than cure. It is most important that those at risk are screened to prevent the disease from transmission to others.

Fortunately the vast majority of people-95% of adults and older children clear the virus spontaneously and develop immunity against it.

Treatment can broadly be divided into 3 stages; **(Management of symptoms, antiviral medication and treatment of advanced liver disease)** as follows:

1. Management of Symptoms

The symptoms of pain, aches and low grade fever should be treated with usual painkillers like Acetaminophen (paracetamol).

Nausea can be managed with anti emetic medication such as Metoclopramide.

There should be regular tests to assess the functions of the liver.

2. Antiviral Medication

There are now potent medications to suppress the virus that cause damage to the liver. Before commencing treatment with these medications, it is important to continually assess the state and functions of the liver by:

- Blood tests
- Liver function tests- alanine aminotransferase- a liver enzyme, and also hepatitis B DNA levels are important markers of liver damage.
- Ultrasound or a fibro scan
- Liver biopsy if found necessary at this stage can be carried out by a specialist in liver disease (hepatologist).

Liver biopsy should assess the degree of damage to the liver by the virus.

In many cases the individual's immune system is able to suppress the virus and prevent any damage to the liver, whilst in others, the damage would be evident and continuous.

In normal functioning liver the drug (**peg interferon alfa 2-a**) is the first line of treatment.

When the liver shows signs of failing, or the above medication is unsuitable, the specialist may resort to antiviral medications such as **tenofovir**.

A good response to the medication would be shown in improvement in health and liver function tests and the specialist may then discontinue the medication.

However, it would be premature and dangerous to stop taking the medication as prescribed even when there appears to be improvement or there are intolerable side effects. Self-assessed discontinuation of treatment could lead to drug resistance and more liver damage. The specialist is therefore the only person to make the decision to continue or discontinue medication.

Peg interferon alfa 2-a is usually used in the treatment of Hepatitis B where there are very high levels of the virus. Its main job is to stimulate the body's natural immune system to fight the virus and regain overall control.

This medication is in injectable form and is given weekly over 12 months. The specialist would then normally conduct tests at 3 and 6 months to assess the effectiveness of medication and the response. Adjustments or outright change to other antiviral medication can then be effected.

Unpleasant side effects such as high temperature, flu-like symptoms and muscle pains are not uncommonly encountered at the commencement of this medication. Normal painkillers such as Acetaminophen (Paracetamol) should be prescribed.

Unfortunately, some people continue to experience quite unpleasant side effects which make the discontinuation of this medication inevitable and so the change to other antiviral medication becomes necessary. These are:

Tenofovir which is in tablet form and should be taken with food and may also cause certain side effects as follows:

- Nausea
- Vomiting
- Diarrhoea
- Tiredness
- Skin rash

- Dizziness

Entecavir is also in tablet form and may have the following side effects:

- Nausea
- Vomiting
- Dizziness
- Sleep problems (insomnia)

Both medications may cause kidney problems and renal function tests should be carried out but the worst side effect is **lactic acidosis** which is the build -up of lactic acid in the blood which can have quite serious consequences in relation to acid- base balance and effects on proper functioning of body systems.

The following symptoms may suggest the possibility of this complication:

- Tiredness
- Weakness
- Breathing difficulties
- Muscle pains
- Coldness of the extremities - the arms and legs
- Nausea with stomach pains
- Dizziness
- Fast or irregular pulse

It is important to contact your specialist as soon as possible if you are on any of these 2 medications and experience some of these warning signs which may be indicative of lactic acidosis and requires urgent management.

The world Health Organization (WHO) recommends the combination of tenofovir and entecavir especially for those with cirrhosis who are at serious risk of liver failure or the development of cancer of the liver.

Treatment of advanced liver disease

The complications of chronic hepatitis infection are **cirrhosis of the liver** and **hepatocellular carcinoma** (cancer of the liver).

Liver function tests and in particular a liver biopsy should be carried out to ascertain when these stages have been reached which usually follow prolonged chronic hepatitis infection.

At these stages of disease, the liver specialist (hepatologist) would have taken over. The above antiviral drugs have already been discussed for the treatment hepatitis B with cirrhosis.

The specialist would normally consider a number of options in the management of liver cancer which would depend on the stage, the extent of spread, the underlying cause, age of the patient and life expectancy.

These options may include:

1. Chemotherapy
2. Surgical resection to remove a diseased section of the liver
3. Transcatheter arterial chemoembolisation (TACE) is another type of chemotherapy used in stages B and C liver cancer. A fine tube is inserted into the femoral artery in the groin and passed to the hepatic artery (the main vessel that carries blood to the

liver). Some chemotherapy medication is then injected directly through the tube into the liver via the blood vessels which supply the cancer cells. This helps to slow down the growth of the cancer cells. Small plastic beads or gel injected during this process help in slowing down the growth of the cancer cells as well by blocking and interfering in their blood supply.
4. Microwave or radiofrequency ablation - where these waves are used to destroy the cancerous cells.
5. Liver transplant.-removing the diseased liver and replacing it with the liver of a healthy donor.
6. Medication called **Sorafenib** can help prolong life. The medication which is given in tablet form interrupts the blood supply to the cancer cells and slows down their growth.
7. This is not routinely available in the UK national Health service as the National Institute for Health and Care Excellence (NICE)considers the cost to outweigh the potential benefit.
8. In advanced disease, only symptomatic treatment to relieve pain , nausea, vomiting, dehydration and the provision of adequate nutrition is usually possible.

PELVIC INFLAMMATORY DISEASE (PID)

This is usually due to infection of the female upper genital tract which may include the fallopian tubes, ovaries and the womb.

Although pelvic inflammatory disease is considered under sexually transmitted infections or disease (STI or STD), in actual fact, only about 25 % are due to this cause. When Pelvic inflammatory Disease (PID) is due to sexually transmitted infections(STI) it is usually due to **Chlamydia** and **gonorrhoea** which spread upwards to involve the womb, fallopian tube and the ovaries.

The remaining cases of PID, 75% are caused by bacteria that normally live in the female genital tract especially the vagina which spread upwards to involve the upper structures above and cause PID. It is not entirely clear why the normal vaginal flora would sometimes become antagonistic to the host and spread upwards to infect the above structures. However, certain factors that cause the lowering of resistance or immunity may play a part. There may also be chemical, hormonal or possibly mechanical factors that play a part in this pathological process.

Symptoms of Pelvic inflammatory Disease

These may be subtle and include any of the following :

1. Lower abdominal or pelvic pain
2. Pain on passing urine (dysuria)
3. Pain between periods (inter menstrual pain)
4. Pain during sexual intercourse especially deeply in the pelvic region (dyspareunia)
5. Pain after sexual intercourse
6. Heavy menstruation (menorrhagia)
7. Painful periods (dysmenorrhoea)
8. Vaginal discharge which may be unusual in quantity especially if green or yellowish in colour.
9. Some women may also experience the following:
10. High temperature.
11. Severe abdominal pain
12. Nausea
13. vomiting

The important clinical implication of pelvic inflammatory disease is the **blockage of the fallopian tube** through inflammation, scarring, narrowing or stricture, thus preventing fertilization of the egg and the transport to the uterus. The consequence here may be **infertility** which has severe implications. Secondly, it may result in **ectopic pregnancy** where the pregnancy actually occurs in some part of the female genital tract instead of the womb; in this case usually the fallopian tube.

It is estimated that about 10% of women who have had pelvic inflammatory disease become infertile but if the condition was recognised and treated early the infertility could be averted.

Recurrent episodes of pelvic inflammatory disease are not uncommon for the following reasons:

1. Failure to complete the course of antibiotics prescribed by the doctor
2. Resistance of the bacterial organisms to the antibiotics prescribed especially where a thorough culture and sensitivity test was not carried out
3. Re-infection by the bacterial flora in the female genital tract.
4. Very importantly, failure to treat the male partner who could then re-infect female partner.
5. Damaged wombs or fallopian tubes are more susceptible to improperly treated infections.

Women with recurrent episodes of pelvic inflammatory disease are more prone to infertility than those who have had only a single well treated episode.

Complications of Pelvic inflammatory disease can be summarised as follow:

1. Abscesses- which is a collection of infected fluid (pus) especially in the fallopian tube, ovary or

adjoining peritoneum. Treatment may involve a combination of antibiotics and/or surgical drainage . Laparoscopic surgery (key hole surgery) may be the best option in experienced hands.
2. Infertility already mentioned above. Possibility of in vivo or even in vitro fertilisation (IVF) should be considered.
3. Ectopic pregnancy -see above. Usually requires surgical intervention to prevent rupture and torrential bleeding. When rupture has already occurred, emergency surgical intervention is required to stop bleeding and save life.
4. Chronic Pain around the lower abdomen and pelvis. Pain should be controlled by normal or strong pain killers.
5. Insomnia (lack of sleep). This can be managed by psychological support and medication in severe cases.
6. Depression especially in chronic or recurrent cases. See management in 5 above.

Prevention of Pelvic Inflammatory Disease

- Use of condoms especially with new partners who have not been tested for STI.
- Have yourself tested for sexually transmitted infections if there is any cause for concern.
- Early treatment of STI
- Early treatment of PID to prevent chronicity and recurrence
- To prevent recurrence, your partner should be tested and treated as necessary.
- Have a check up for STI before any surgical/gynaecological manipulations around the uterus, cervix or vagina, such as coil insertion or abortion as any of these may precipitate ascending infection.

Dr. Usen Ikidde

Treatment of Pelvic inflammatory Disease

Pelvic Inflammatory infections can easily be treated by antibiotics. It is important to recognise the symptoms of PID and tell your doctor or be referred to a specialist clinic. In many cases family doctors can usually prescribe suitable antibiotics without the need for referral. Antibiotic treatment is usually a combination to take care of the most likely infections such as Chlamydia and gonorrhoea. In addition to these, there are a number of gram negative bacteria which also have to be considered as possible cause of PID infection and so have to be treated as well. In some cases a cervical swab and sensitivity may be carried out especially if the symptoms continue despite treatment.

Pregnancy should be excluded before certain antibiotics are prescribed. It is therefore important to tell your doctor if you think you might be pregnant.

In order to clear PID infection, a longer course, 14 days of a combination of antibiotics is usually prescribed. Patients are strongly advised to complete the course of the antibiotics to prevent recurrence, antibiotic resistance, complications and chronicity of infection.

A combination of the following or similar antibiotics are usually prescribed:

- Metronidazole for gram negative bacteria
- Doxycycline
- Ofloxacin
- Ceftriaxone

Treatment may often consist of injection as well as tablets. Severe cases of PID should usually have antibiotics through a drip (intravenous antibiotics).

Painkillers should also be given as some patients may experience severe pain which requires careful consideration and treatment.

A follow up appointment may be necessary to assess whether the prescribed antibiotics are working as expected in relieving symptoms. Such follow up appointment should be arranged on the third day after starting treatment.

LYMPHOGRANULOMA VENEREUM (LGV)

Lymphogranuloma Venereum is a sexually transmitted disease caused by **Chlamydia trachomatis** bacterium.

You would have noticed that this is the same bacterium that causes Chlamydia and trachoma and may also be responsible for non-**gonococcal urethritis**, cervicitis, salpingitis, pneumonia and pelvic inflammatory disease.

It may usually first be noticed by the characteristic enlargement of the lymph nodes of the groin as LGV is primarily an infection of lymphatics and lymph nodes. The LGV bacteria normally travel to the lymph nodes of the groin through a break in the skin or via the epithelium of the mucous membrane.

The infection may take up to 3-30 days after the initial contact with the bacteria to manifest in the lymph nodes.

Infection is usually acquired by sexual contact through the following:

External sex organs-

1. The penis

2. The vagina
3. The anus -which it may cause proctitis or proctocolitis (Inflammation of the ano-rectal region or the rectum and large intestine).

The initial appearance in the male may be as a painless genital ulcer on the penis but in the female this may not be visible as the ulcer occurs inside the vagina and is hidden from view.

The diagnosis is usually by a serological test which is by complement fixation test. The clinical manifestation of LGV is an ulcer on the genital areas or enlarged lymph nodes of the groin. These would point to the possibility of LGV and the test should be carried out to ascertain the diagnosis.

Until 2003 LGV was regarded as rare in the developed countries. However, in that year, an outbreak occurred in male homosexual population in the Netherlands. Since then several cases have been reported in other European countries-Germany, UK, France, Italy, Switzerland, Belgium, and Sweden. There have also been reports in the US and Canada. These new cases were a newly discovered variant of the bacteria which was the same variant (L2b) that was found in Amsterdam (Netherlands) in 2003. They were also associated with gay men.

Prevention

These include:

1. Early diagnosis and treatment based on symptoms especially in male homosexual community.
2. The use of condoms

3. Avoidance of sexual contact with infected people until they have been tested, treated and declared infection- free.

Treatment

Tetracycline is the antibiotic of choice but this antibiotic is contraindicated in pregnancy. The bacteria also respond to Erythromycin.

This is another disease which its resurgence may be of interest to the World Health Organization (WHO) and which appropriate and effective preventive and therapeutic measures should be instituted to eradicate the infection and stop the spread.

CHANCROID

Chancroid is a sexually transmitted disease (STD) caused by the bacteria Haemophilus ducreyi.

The disease is found mainly in developing countries and spread mostly by prostitution and is prevalent in poor societies. In many developed economies, socio- economic group may not be such an important factor as it is in third world countries.

It is characterised by causing **painful ulcers** on the genital organs in the following areas:

In men-

1. The shaft of the penis
2. The Glans penis
3. The corona of the penis
4. Urethral opening

5. The foreskin
6. The inner thighs

In women-

1. The vagina where there may be as many as 4 or more sores or ulcers
2. The labia majora-often "kissing ulcers" that occur on the opposite sides.
3. The labia minora
4. The clitoris
5. The inner thigh
6. The perianal region

The clinical features may consist of the following:

1. Painful sore or ulcer on any of the sites above
2. The ulcers have ragged irregular or sharply defined borders.
3. The base of the ulcer is covered by yellowish material.
4. Bleeding of the base can occur especially when traumatized.
5. Pain on passing urine (dysuria)
6. Pain on sexual intercourse (dyspareunia) especially in the female.
7. Painful enlarged lymph nodes of the groin (lymphadenopathy).

It is important to distinguish Syphilitic ulcer (chancre) from chancroid ulcer.

The most important differences to note are as follows:

1. Syphilitic ulcer is typically painless whilst chancroid ulcer is painful.

2. Syphilitic ulcer does not usually produce any exudate (fluid) at the base whereas chancroid produces yellowish exudative purulent (like pus) material at the base.
3. Syphilitic ulcers have hard raised edges whilst Chancroid ulcers typically have soft edges.
4. Syphilitic ulcers heal spontaneously in about 4-6 weeks whereas Chancroid ulcers may take much longer time to heal.
5. Syphilitic ulcers may occur in the pharynx as well as the genital area whereas Chancroid ulcers occur mostly in the genital areas.

Prevention

1. Prevention may be helped by the use of condom but this does not entirely eliminate transmission as leakage of fluid exudate can still occur freely around the genital uncovered areas.
2. Avoid sexual contact with people who have not been tested.
3. Holiday makers should avoid unprotected or protected sexual activities with the local population especially with commercial sex workers.
4. Early treatment of ulcers and avoidance of sexual contact until declared disease-free should be the norm.

Treatment.

Antibiotics are usually effective as follows:

1. Oral Erythromycin for 7 days or
2. A single oral dose of 1gm of Azithromycin or
3. A single intramuscular injection of Cetriazone.

The physician will usually check for contraindication of any antibiotic during pregnancy.

MOLLUSCUM CONTAGIOSUM

This is a highly contagious viral infection of the skin which occurs at any age especially in children aged 1-10 years. It is caused by Molluscum contagiosum virus(MCV).

There are 4 types of the virus-MCV-1 to-4. The most prevalent is MCV-1, but MCV-2 is the type mostly found in adults.

Molluscum Contagiosum is considered under sexually transmitted infections despite only about a quarter(25%) being due to this cause.

The infection is spread chiefly through the following routes:

1. Close direct contact with infected person
2. Sharing of infected objects such as clothes, underwear, towels and toys
3. Sexual contact which may be in the form of close physical intimacy or actual sexual intercourse.
4. Autoinoculation of the same person which involves contact of infected part of the body with non-infected part thereby transferring infection to that part. Alternatively, infection of a different part of the body can be effected by touching the infected part and inadvertently transferring it to a different part.

Infection by MC continues as long as the spots remain. The central waxy core contains the virus and spreads to other parts of the body as in number 4 above by direct or indirect contact.

The **symptoms** are usually as follows:

1. Raised spots on the skin which may vary in size from about 1-10 mm.in diameter.
2. The spots are usually red or pink in colour with tiny whitish yellow head in the centre.
3. Rupture of the spot releases a thick whitish or yellowish highly infectious material which is infectious to others or capable of causing autoinoculation.
4. There is a tendency for spread to other parts of the body to occur and so with time the spots are not confined to a single anatomical part of the body. Such spread is typical of MC and should be suspected from the nature and characteristic of the spots described above.
5. The spots are usually painless unless bacterial infection has supervened with inflammation which causes pain.
6. The spots may be itchy especially if there are areas of dry, cracked, or reddish skin around them.

The spots could affect most parts of the body especially the following:

1. Trunk
2. Face
3. Neck
4. Upper and lower limbs
5. Genitals and surrounding areas especially if spread is by sexual contact.

The spots tend to crust and heal spontaneously within 2-3 months and leave a light skin or pitted mark rather than scars. In other cases they clear up in less than a year but occasionally persist for many years especially if:

1. The spots break up and infect other parts of the body (autoinoculation).
2. When the individual affected has a weakened immunity.
3. Persistent sexual intimacy with infected partner in which re-infection may occur.
4. In HIV infection
5. Patients on chemotherapy

Prevention

1. Avoid skin to skin contact with infected person.
2. Avoid the sharing of items of clothing and also towels.
3. There should be no sexual contact with infected partner until declared infection-free.
4. Minimise autoinoculation if at all possible in order to reduce duration and area of infection.

Treatment

There is no absolute certainty that treatment does any good except in complicated cases. This is because the spots normally disappear spontaneously.

The following topical applications may sometimes be found useful:

1. Potassium Hydroxide applied twice daily.
2. Podophyllotoxin-This poisons the cells of the spot. The correct dosage should be drawn up by a special applicator and applied to each spot.

3. **Imiquimod** is used for larger spots to stimulate the immune system to attack the infection . The cream is applied to the spots and washed off in 6-8 hours and used 3 times weekly.

Unfortunately, two large randomized controlled trials in the US completed in 2006 demonstrated that after 18 weeks of application that the treatment was not superior to a placebo.

In addition to this, Imiquimod cream has several undesirable side effects such as:

1. Erythema
2. scabbing and crusting of the skin
3. scaling and flaking of the skin
4. otitis media especially in adults
5. conjunctivitis
6. oedema
7. erosion of the skin
8. weeping of the skin
9. Systemic absorption of the cream could have negative effect on white blood cell count.
10. itching of the skin
11. Burning sensation
12. May cause headache in some patients.

Benzoyl Peroxide

This is usually applied to the spots 1-2 times daily. The area should be washed and dried before application of the cream or gel. It should be used sparingly to avoid injury to the skin.

There may still be the following side effects:

1. burning sensation
2. itching
3. dryness and redness of the skin
4. increased sensitivity to sunlight.
5. peeling of the skin

Surgical Treatment

1. **Cryotherapy-** involves freezing the spots with liquid nitrogen for 5-10 seconds and may require several sessions to clear the spots completely. Cryotherapy should be carried out at intervals of 2-3 times a week.
2. **Diathermy** uses heat to remove the spots after applying some local anaesthetic to prevent pain.
3. **Curettage.**

A curette is used to scrape off the spots. A local anaesthetic agent is applied to prevent pain that may be experienced during this procedure.

4. **Pulsed-dye laser.**

Laser treatment involves the use of a powerful beam of light to destroy the cells of the spot. It may need to be repeated several times before the spots are fully cleared. This treatment may cause skin discolouration and some discomfort.

CHAPTER SIX

NEGLECTED TROPICAL DISEASEs

Concerns had been expressed over the years about certain tropical diseases which appeared forgotten or neglected.The World Health Organization (WHO)stepped in to address the concerns in kind and in cash. It officially declared 17 "Neglected Tropical Diseases"(NTD).

Neglected Tropical Diseases impact on the lives of over 1billion people in 149 countries world wide. NTD are associated with poverty and low socio-economic status.They are mostly concentrated in rural or urban slums. Those affected by NTD are usually those individuals and communities who are, by their circumstances, unable to vocalize or articulate their problems in political circles.

NTD are associated with suffering,chronic or life long disability, distress sometimes stigmatization,discrimination and mental distress.

Fortunately, the WHO has now come to the rescue of these communities with a view to the elimination of these diseases.

The WHO in keeping with its policy has decided to adopt an integrated intervention -centred approach with a focus on marginalized and poor communities with one or more these five interventional public health approaches:

1. Preventive chemotherapy
2. Intensified Case Management
3. Vector Control
4. Veterinary Public Health
5. Safe Water,Sanitation and Hygiene.

The WHO effort has been complemented and supplemented by various bodies, institutions and Organizations.Some pharmaceutical companies have donated medications. There have been innovative research in new methods of treatment, prevention and new diagnostic tools.Ministries of Health in affected countries have largely implemented the WHO integrated initiatives to help combat these diseases and support the global network of both highly motivated private and public bodies.

Lately, Bill Gates and his wife,Melinda, have thrown their full weights behind the WHO initiative and founded the "Bill and Melinda Gates Foundation" to help tackle the NTD.

The WHO, in a summary publication issued the following statement about the 17 Neglected Tropical Diseases.

Neglected Tropical Diseases-Summary:

1. "**Dengue**:a mosquito-borne-infection causing flu-like illness that may develop into severe dengue and cause lethal complications.
2. **Rabies:**A preventable viral diseases transmitted to humans through the bites of dogs that is invariably fatal once symptoms develop.
3. **Trachoma:** A Chlamydial infction transmitted through direct contact with infectious eye or nasal discharge, or through indirect contact with unsafe living conditions and hygiene practices, which left

untreated causes irreversible corneal opacities and blindness.
4. **Buruli ulcer:** A debilitating mycobacterium skin infection causing severe destruction of the skin, bone and soft tissue.
5. **Yaws:** A chronic bacterial infection affecting mainly the skin and bone.
6. **Leprosy:** A complex disease caused by infection mainly of the skin, peripheral nerves, mucosa of the upper respiratory tract and eyes.
7. **Chagas Disease:** A life-threatening illness transmitted to humans through contact with vector insects (triatomine bugs), ingestion of contaminated food, infected blood transfusions, congenital transmission, organ transplantation or laboratory accidents.
8. **Human African Trypanosomiasis (Sleeping Sickness)**: A parasitic infection spread by the bites of tsetse flies that is almost 100% fatal without prompt diagnosis and treatment to prevent the parasites invading the central nervous system.
9. .**Leishmaniasis**: Disease transmitted through the bites of infected female sandflies that in its most severe (visceral) form attacks the internal organs and in its most prevalent (cutaneous) form causes face ulcers, disfiguring scars and disability.
10. **Taeniasis and neurocysticercosis:** An infection caused by adult tapeworm in human intestines; cysticercosis results when humans ingest tapeworm eggs that develop as larvae in tisues.
11. **Drancunculiasis (guinea -worm diseases)**: A nematode infection transmitted exclusively by drinking-water contaminated with parasite-infected water fleas.
12. **Echinococcosis**: Infection caused by the larval stages of tapeworms forming pathogenic cysts in

humans and transmitted when ingesting eggs most commonly shed in faeces of dogs and wild animals.
13. **Foodborne trematodiasis:** Infection acquired by consuming fish, vegetables and crustaceans contaminated by larval parasites; clonochiasis, opisthorchiasis and fascioliasis are the main diseases.
14. **Lymphatic filariasis**: Infection transmitted by mosquitoes causing abnormal enlargement of limbs and genitals from adult worms inhabiting and reproducing in the lymphatic system.
15. **Onchocerciasis (river blindness):** Infection transmitted by the bite of infected blackflies causing severe itching and eye lesions as the adult worm produces lavae and leading to visual impairment and permanent blindness.
16. **Schistosomiasis**: Trematode infections transmitted when larval forms released by freshwater snails penetrate human skin during contact with infested water.
17. **Soil- transmitted helminthiasis**: Nematode infections transmitted through soil contaminated by human faeces causing anaemia, vitamin A deficiency, stunted growth, malnutrition intestinal obstruction and impaired development".

REFERENCES

1. British National Formulary (September 2014-March 2015 ed.68).BMJ Group and the Royal Society of Great Britain.
2. Immunization Against Infectious Diseases (2006).www.immunization. dh.gov.uk.
3. Public Health England-Policies,Publications,Consultations,Statistics.22nd June 2015
4. Dirckx, J. (1997).Steadman's Concise Medical & Allied Health Dictionary. Baltimore. Philadelphia. London. Paris: Williams & Wilkins.
5. Public Health England,10 September 2015.
6. NHS Choices,Your Health,Your Choices.
7. Wikepedia.Org/wiki/malaria,tuberculosis,yellow fever,hepatitis,typhoid,cholera,dipheria,poliomyelitis ,Ebola,Japanese Encephalitis,tick-borne encephalitis,Lassa fever,Chickenpox,influenza virus, measles, African Trypanosomiasis, Avian flu, dengue, hand, foot and mouth disease,leptospirosis,meningococcal disease,mumps,Murray valley encephalitis virus,pneumococcal disease,rabies,Rift valley fever,rubella,scabies,schistosomiasis,tetanus,west nile virus,Middle East respiratory syndrome,Zika virus, immunization, sexually transmitted diseases.
8. WHO media center.
9. Ikidde, U.(2014) Beat constipation without laxatives and lose weight that is sustainable and permanent.Bloomington:Author House.
10. NICE guidelines Anti D Immunoglobulin.

11. Ryan, E. T. Kain, K. C.(2000) Health Advice and Immunization for Travellers,New England Journal.Med.
12. World Health Organization (1996).The State Of World Health: World Health Report:Fighting Disease,fostering development.Geneva 1997,p 1-62.
13. Matteli, A.Carosi,G.(2001)Sexually Transmitted Diseases in Travellers:Sexually Infect.Dis.2001:1063-7.
14. Gerbase,A.C.Rowley,J.T.Mertens,T. E.(1998).Globally Epidemiology of Sexually Transmitted Diseases,Lancet 1998:351 (Suppl 3):2-41016/S0140-6736(98)-0 (PubMed).
15. World Health Organization/Global Program on AIDS.Global Prevalence and Incidence Estimates of Selected curable sexually transmitted diseases: Overview and estimates.Geneva Organization.1995;1-26.
16. Etkind P, Ratelle S.Harvey, G. (2003). International Travel and Sexually Transmitted Disease.9(2) :1654-1656.Emerg.Infect Dis .2003 Dec 9 (12):1654-1656.
17. Center for Disease Control (CDC) and Prevention. CDC 24/7 :Saving Lives ,Protecting People.
18. Public Health England:Malaria:guidance data analysis.Advisory Committee on malaria Prevention (ACMP) 11th September 2015.
19. Peters, W. Giles, H. M. Tropical Medicine & Parasitology.Wolfe Medical Publishing Ltd .London.
20. Netdoctor.co.uk
21. Center for Disease Control (1982) "Update on on Acquired Immune Deficiency Syndrome (AIDS) - United States".MMWR Morb Mortal Wkly Rep31 (37) :507-508;513-514.PMID 6815471.
22. Sharp P. M, Hahn B.H(2011) "Origins Of HIV and the AIDS Pandemic. Cold Spring Habor Perspectives in Medicine 1(9)

a006841.doi:1101/cshper.a006841.pmc3234451.PMID22229120.
23. Zhn, T. Korber, B.T.Nahmias,AJ.Hooper, E,Sharp, P.M.Ho, DD(1998)"An African HIV-1 Sequence from 1959 and implications for the origin of the epidemic".Nature 391(6667):594-7.Bibcode:1998 Nature .391.594Z.doi:10.1038/35400 PMID 9468138.
24. Kolata, G. (October 28 1987)."Boys 1969 death suggests AID invaded US several times" .The New York Times.
25. Kleinman, S.(September 2004).Patient Information :Blood donation and Transfusion Update.Archived Information.
26. Servile, M.(2012),Medical Entomology for students (5th edition). Cambridge University Press 1SB978-1-10766818-8.
27. Centre for Disease Control and Prevention (2 November 2010). Parasites-Scabies Treatment.
28. World Health Organization (WHO) .Water Related Diseases.
29. World Health Organization (WHO).Scabies.
30. International Alliance For the Control Of Scabies.
31. World Health Organization (WHO).Neglected Tropical Diseases.
32. World Health Organization (WHO) "The 17 Neglected Tropical Diseases.
33. Center For Disease Control and Prevention CDC (October 2004) "Lymphogranuloma Venereum among men who have sex with men-Netherlands 2003-2004"MMMR Morb Mortality wkly.Rep53(42)985-8 PMD 15514580.
34. Current Diagnosis and Treatment of Sexually Transmitted Diseases.MCGraw-Hill Companies Inc 2007.PP69-74,ISBN 9780071509619.
35. American Academy of Dermatology(2006)

Pamplets:Molluscum Contagiosum.

36. Center for Disease Control and Prevention (2013)."Molluscum Contagiosum"
37. Avian Influenza A (H5N1) Infection in Humans by Writing Committee of the World Health Organization (WHO) Consultation on Human Influenza A/H5 In September 29,2005.New England Journal of Medicine.
38. "Hand,Foot and Mouth Disease: Signs and Symptoms". Myoclinic.com
39. World Health Organization (2006).Avian Influenza ("bird flu")-The Disease in Humans.
40. Reiter, P.(11 March 2010) "Yellow Fever and Dengue: a threat to Europe?".Euro Surveill 15 (10) 19509.
41. Global Strategy For Dengue Prevention and Control (PDF) World Health Organization 2012. P16-17.ISBN978-92-4-150403-4.
42. Hand Foot and Mouth Disease: Prevention and Treatment.Center For Disease Control and Prevention 2013.
43. China reports 537 deaths from hand-foot-mouth disease this year. People's Daily on line 2010.
44. Health Ministry :Hand -foot-mouth Disease claims 50 lives this year. China View.10 April 2009.
45. Bacterial Meningitis and meningococcal Septicaemia :management of bacterial septicaemia in children and people younger than 16 years in primary and secondary care ;NICE Clinical Guidelines (June 2010).
46. Meningococcal:the green book,chapter 22;Public Health England (July 2015).
47. Meningococcal:ACWY Programme; information for healthcare professionals;Public Health England ,8 July 2015.

48. Ryan, K. J.Ray, C.G. (2004) Sheris Medical Microbiology.McGraw Hill. ISBN 0-8385-8529-9.
49. Rabies Fact Sheet: World Health Organization July 2013.
50. WHO Expert Consultation on Rabies: Second Report. Geneva :WHO 2013.
51. Symptoms of rabies: NHS.uk .June 12,2012.
52. Rabies: AnimalsWeCare .com
53. www.thecattlesite.com/disease info/254/rift valley-fever.
54. Rift Valley Fever-The Center for Food Security and Public. Health. Infections Enzootic Hepatitis of Sheep and Cattle .Updated January 2015.
55. Palmer, S.R (2011) Oxford Textbook Of Zooneses :biology,clinical practice and Public Health Control (2nd ed) Oxford University Press.
56. Rift Valley Fever:Wikipedia,the free Encyclopedia.
57. World Health Organization (WHO) Fact Sheet. Schistosomiasis. Updated February 2016.
58. World Health Organization (WHO).Neglected Tropical Diseases-Summary (Fact Sheet).
59. Tetanus Causes and Transmission .www.cdc.gov January 9,2013.
60. Tetanus-Symptoms and Complications. cdc.gov. January 9,2013.
61. Tetanus For Clinicians. Cdc.gov.January 2013.
62. Elimination of Maternal and Neonatal Tetanus. 7 July 2015.UNICEF.Retrieved 4 April 2016.
63. Hayes, E.B.Komar, N.Nasci, R. S.Montgomery, S. P. O'Leary D R.Campbell, G L , (2005) "Epidemiology and Transmission Dynamics Of West Nile Virus Disease" Emerging Infec.Disease 11(8) 1167-73.
64. Oklahoma State University :Mosquitoes and West Nile Virus.
65. Watson, J.T. Pertel, P.E. Jones, R. C et al (September 2014)."Clinical Characteristics and

Functional Outcomes of West Nile Fever.Ann.Intern.Med.
66. "Mosquito Monitoring and Management". National Park Service.
67. World Health Organization (WHO).West Nile Virus .Factsheet fs 354/en/.
68. Middle East Respiratory Syndrome Corona virus (MERS-CoV)-"Saudi Arabia".World Health Organization.11 June 2015.
69. "MERS death count up to 29" HiDoc.25 June 2015.
70. "Middle East Respiratory Syndrome Coronavirus (MERS-CoV).Summary and Literature update-as of 20 January 2014"(PDF)World Health Organization 20 January 2014.
71. Interim Guidance -Clinical Management of severe acute respiratory infections when novel coronavirus is suspected :"What to do and what not to do"WHO 2 November 2013.
72. Daniel, K. W. Chu, Leo L. M. Mokhtar, M. etal (Volume 20,Number 6-June 2014) MERS corona virus in Dromedary Carmels,Egypt.
73. "Middle East Respiratory Syndrome Corona virus (MERS-CoV) -Saudi Arabia".WHO Updates 14 April 2016.
74. Middle East Respiratory Syndrome Corona virus (MERS-CoV) -Republic of Korea.24 May2015.
75. Middle East Respiratory Syndrome Corona virus (Mers-Cov)-China 31 May 2015.
76. "Novel Coronavirus update-new virus to be called MERS-CoV"(Press Release).WHO.15 May 2013.Retrieved 20 April 2016.
77. "Novel Corona virus infection" (Press Release) WHO.25 September 2012.Retrieved 20 April 2016.
78. "Global Alert and Response (GAR).Novel Corona virus Infection -Update"(Press Release) WHO.23 November 2012.Retrieved 20 April 2016.

79. Otromke John, et al (20 October 2014).Investigating Treatment Strategies for the Middle East Respiratory Syndrome Coronavirus".The Pharmaceutical Journal 293.Retrieved 20 April 2016.
80. "Middle East Respiratory Syndrome Corona virus (MERS-CoV) -Turkey".World Health Organization.24 October 2014. Retrieved 20 April 2016.
81. "Coronavirus never before seen in humans is the cause of SARS".United Nations World Health Organization.16 April 2006.Retrieved 25 April 2016.
82. "Scientists prove SARS -civet cat link".China Daily.23 November 2006. Retrieved 25 April 2016.
83. World Health Organization (WHO) .Zika Virus Fact Sheet. 15 April 2016. Accessed 26 April 2016.
84. World Health Organization (WHO) "Guillain Barre Syndrome". Fact Sheet. 14 March 2016.Accessed 26 April 2016.
85. Unitednaija. "Woman in Kaduna gave birth to half Human half Donkey".Press Report 24 January 2016.Retrieved 28 April 2016.
86. Nairaland Forum."Human in Kaduna gave birth to half Human half Donkey". 24 January 2016.Press Report. Accessed 28 April 2016.
87. New England Journal of Medicine (May 2016).Zika Virus Birth Defects May Be Tip of the Iceberg". Experts say.Maggie Fox Report. Press Release. Accessed 2 May 2016
88. "Zika Virus Microcephaly and Guillain-Barre Syndrome Situation Report".World Health Organization. 7 April 2016.Retrieved 2 May 2016.
89. Zika Virus in the Caribbean. "Travellers' Health:Travel Notices. Center For Disease Control and Prevention.15 January 2016. Retrieved 2 May 2016.

90. "Zika Virus Infection Outbreak,Brazil and the Pacific Region"(PDF).Rapid Risk Assessment.Stockholm: European Centre for Disease Prevention and Control 25 May 2016.
91. Chastain, Mary. (30 January 2016)"National Institute Of Health: Zika Virus is a Pandemic".Retrieved 2 May 2016.
92. "Zika Virus: Advice for planning to travel to outbreak areas".ITV Report (ITV News) 22 January 2016.Accessed 2 May 2016.
93. "For Health Care Providers:Clinical Evaluation and Disease".Zika Virus.Center For Disease Control and Prevention .19 January 2016.Retrieved 2 May 2016.
94. Zika Virus in the United States 2015-2016". Center For Disease Control and Prevention.27 April 2016.Accessed 2 May 2016.
95. Zika Virus(3 March 2016)."Symptoms, Diagnosis and Treatment".Center For Disease Control and Prevention.Atlanta.Accessed 4 May 2016.
96. World Health Organization (WHO) (22 November 2015). "Neglected Tropical Diseases Summary".
97. World Health Health Organization (WHO) (2012."Accelerating Work to overcome the global impact of Neglected Tropical Diseases.A Road Map for Implementation". Geneva,Switzerland.
98. World Health Organization WHO (24 November 2015). "Neglected Tropical Diseases".

www.ingramcontent.com/pod-product-compliance
Lightning Source LLC
Chambersburg PA
CBHW071414180526
45170CB00001B/100